SUGAR COATING
DIABETES

The Empowering Truth About Diet, Supplements, and Drugs

ED POSNAK

Note for Librarians: A cataloguing record for this book is available from Library and Archives Canada at www.collectionscanada.ca/amicus/index-e.html
ISBN 1-4120-8353-2

Printed on paper with minimum 30% recycled fibre. Trafford's print shop runs on "green energy" from solar, wind and other environmentally-friendly power sources.

TRAFFORD
PUBLISHING

Offices in Canada, USA, Ireland and UK

Book sales for North America and international:
Trafford Publishing, 6E–2333 Government St.,
Victoria, BC V8T 4P4 CANADA
phone 250 383 6864 (toll-free 1 888 232 4444)
fax 250 383 6804; email to orders@trafford.com
Book sales in Europe:
Trafford Publishing (UK) Limited, 9 Park End Street, 2nd Floor
Oxford, UK OX1 1HH UNITED KINGDOM
phone 44 (0)1865 722 113 (local rate 0845 230 9601)
facsimile 44 (0)1865 722 868; info.uk@trafford.com
Order online at:
trafford.com/ 06-0108

10 9 8 7 6

Table of Contents

Acknowledgements

Several people have contributed in one form or another to *Sugarcoating Diabetes*. I would like to thank the following people for their contributions:

George Posnak, who not only reviewed several full drafts of the manuscript, but who, through our numerous discussions, simultaneously challenged and inspired my ideas.

Reviewers Anita Simons and Melissa Bolthouse for their encouragement and detailed feedback on several early drafts; Brahm Windeler for his thorough and detailed reviews of multiple drafts; Alan Zeleznikar, Andrew McEvoy, Bert Krages II, Betsy Franz, Bob Samuels, Dale Ingmanson, Gretchen Ingmanson, Kevin Hulen, Reverend Bob, Russ Farris, Sally Ingmanson, and Todd Lorenz for their insightful comments and suggestions.

Supporters Susan Cheng for her comments and insights, and for lending me her endocrinology textbooks and papers; John Gebbie for our wine-enhanced discussions that helped me to unveil the core themes of this book; Vanessa Lee, Jeanne Moncada, and Andrew Ziffer for their feedback and encouragement.

Artists Dustin Zahn for an amazing cover layout and Scott Madison for his excellent drawings.

Benevolent ones Adrienne Durso for supplying items pictured on the front cover and for her encouragement; George Settanni for his financial contributions; Cheryl Dodge, for being cool about my photographing product labels at her grocery store; Chris Geen, for recommending the Schwarzbein Principle, which started it all for me; and George Howard, whose life of service inspired this effort.

Disclaimer

The information contained in *Sugarcoating Diabetes* is for educational purposes only and is not meant as a substitute for medical advice or care. The author of this book is not a medical professional or practitioner. The reader should regularly consult a qualified health care professional for medical advice and care.

Preface

This book is different from most books you will find on the subject of diabetes. I, the author, am not a doctor promoting a new diet, miracle cure, or weight loss program. Rather, I am a type 2 diabetic who has discovered that there is a great deal of misinformation about diabetes being circulated and that knowing the truth can save us from a lot of pain and suffering. My goal is to eliminate as much of that pain and suffering as I can by exposing the myths that perpetuate our struggle. As such, *Sugarcoating Diabetes* debunks misinformation with facts, culled from books, medical journals, reports, and court testimonies. Knowing these facts has empowered me to succeed against diabetes and I am inspired to share that knowledge with you.

Sugarcoating Diabetes is not an introductory "Diabetes 101" text for idiots or dummies. Rather, it is a companion text that explains how and why much of the conventional wisdom that often finds its way into such books is misleading or simply wrong. For completeness, all of the terms and concepts used in *Sugarcoating Diabetes* are explained fully in *Appendix A: Diabetes FAQ*. Even if you are already a diabetes expert, I invite you to review this appendix because you might find a few surprises. In keeping with the theme of the book, the appendix debunks sugarcoated myths with facts.

Whether you have diabetes or care for someone who does, *Sugarcoating Diabetes* will reveal to you some interesting facts that may help change your life for the better.

1

Introduction

I remember waiting for the elevator for the doctor's office at St. Jude's hospital. I had to pee so bad I was going to wet my pants, and the elevator was slower than a California DMV employee on Valium. I was dancing around with one leg in the air, my two-liter water bottle in one hand and my laptop bag in the other. I remember how angry I was about wasting my morning waiting in some doctor's office. The strangeness of carrying around a bottle of water everywhere and peeing like a fire hose didn't even enter my thought process.

I could tell by the look in the nurse's face that something was very wrong. She asked me if I had eaten. No, breakfast that day had consisted of Starbucks and a Marlboro light. I didn't know what a fasting plasma glucose of 436 meant, but she explained. Later the doctor performed some more tests. My HbA1c was 12.8—far outside the normal range of 5.4 to 6.4—and my insulin near zero. The doctor diagnosed me and sent me on my way with three drug prescriptions and a bag full of free samples.

In just a few hours, I went from having a normal life (with a 2-liter bottle of water attached at the hip) to one that would be full of medications, finger sticks, hospital visits, waiting rooms, insurance claims, blood tests, support groups, and possibly needles. The thought of needles was enough to motivate me to do everything I could to keep my sugar under control. I quit smoking. I followed the American Diabetes Association dietary guidelines and switched to using sugar-free and low fat products. I took all my medications at the regularly scheduled times. I was thankful for the modern wonders of biotechnology that allowed me to continue working long, stressful hours behind a desk while my diabetes was controlled for me. Except, as my meter frequently reminded me, it wasn't. Despite all the medication and sugar-free maple syrup, my blood sugars kept creeping up.

Could anything be done? "The disease progresses," I was told. Not knowing any better, I continued the medication and ADA diet regimen believing that I was doing everything I could for my diabetes. I had no interest in learning anything more than what my health care team told me. After all, they were the experts.

Then, one day a friend lent me a book that his wife, who had gestational diabetes, had found very helpful. The book, *The Schwarzbein Principle*, taught me some new things about nutrition, but more important, it opened my eyes to a profound realization: *much of what we are led to believe about health is wrong.* This conventional "wisdom" is contradicted by science, yet it appears in books, educational materials, and recommendations from authorities. At the time I didn't understand all the reasons for this, but I was nonetheless intrigued with the possibility that in science there might be a better way to manage diabetes, one that could empower me to overcome my seemingly inevitable fate.

I read all the books on diabetes, health, and nutrition that I could find. Most of the books contained the same basic information about glucose and insulin, etc., but when it came to the subjects of diet, supplements, and medication, viewpoints were all over the map. It was disturbingly unclear whether I was better off eating bacon and eggs or low-fat bran muffins for breakfast. I couldn't tell whether chromium was going to improve my insulin function or just drain my wallet. While some sources claimed oral diabetes medications were a cure-all, others revealed that these drugs were hardly effective, eventually stopped working, and some even had dangerous side effects.

I continued to read incessantly, but became increasingly frustrated with the inconsistency I found. Science, I knew, should be self-consistent. Facts and rigorous logic should always arrive at the same conclusion. However, on the subjects of diet, drugs, and supplements, the writers not only disagreed, they did so passionately. Views were so polarized and partisan that it seemed nutrition and health science more resembled political science than physical science.

Not knowing who to believe, I decided to put to work the scientific research skills I learned as a PhD student and get to the real science underlying all this confusion. I went to the source of the information—the data and studies used to support the various conflicting theories—so that I could get some straight answers. It wasn't long before I came to the following realizations:

1. *there is a lot we don't know about diabetes*

2. *what we do know is not accurately reflected in the media*

3. *money is the root of all this sugarcoating*

The reason for the controversy became clear. Type 2 diabetes is an enormous and growing market, representing billions of dollars annually in the sales of specialty "diet" foods, supplements, prescription drugs, and other diabetes products. Because so much money is riding on what products we consume, millions of dollars are spent annually to influence the daily choices of diabetics and those who treat them. This high powered marketing takes many forms, from the overt ads for "guilt-free" desserts lining the pages of diabetes magazines to the covert sales pitches for drugs disguised as continuing medical education for health professionals.

Today more than ever, doctors, nurses, educators, and patients are fed a steady diet of oversimplified, distorted, and biased information for the purpose of selling products. All of this marketing disguised as education just keeps us stumbling around in the darkness and those of us with diabetes ultimately suffer the consequences. Misinformed and ignorant to the forces at play, we diligently follow baseless advice, spend countless dollars, and get poor results.

The good news is that seeing through the sugarcoating can improve the quality and quantity of your life. Recognizing and discarding misinformation will allow you to make choices based on the best available information. These choices are what will ultimately determine whether you experience the complications of diabetes or lead a complication-free life. Several large-scale studies have demonstrated that positive lifestyle changes, even sub-optimal ones, are more powerful than any drug in preventing diabetes and its complications.[1,2,3]

I have personally experienced the power of making well-informed decisions. By making lifestyle changes based on real science, not "sugarcoated" science fiction, I was able to reverse the progression of my diabetes and now live a normal, healthy life without medication. I don't count grams of carbohydrates or fat and I don't have any other gimmicky secret to success. My secret is a steady diet of sugar-free information that allows me to make effective daily choices. I do not have a quick and easy cure for diabetes, but I have something that works consistently, like the science it is based on.

I believe the facts presented in this book will open your eyes to ideas that can transform your life as they have mine. This transformation requires that we reserve credibility for the facts, and only the facts, so that we can *know* rather than just *believe* what we are told. When it comes to diabetes management, believing isn't good enough anymore. We need facts. I am inspired to share with you the facts I have learned because I believe they can make the critical difference between winning and losing the battle against diabetes. I hope that they make a positive difference in your life.

Part I: Diet

What should I eat if I have diabetes? This is the question we all ask. We know we shouldn't eat what we ate to become diabetic, but that still leaves us with many options. Apples or avocados? Bacon or biscuits? What about low-fat foods? Is low-carb healthy? How many grams of carbs can we have? What percentage of calories should come from fat?

For all of our questions there is no shortage of answers. Indeed, the great thing about the diabetic diet is that there are so many to choose from. Atkins is a popular one these days. Then you have Dr. Phil, The Zone, South Beach, Sugar Busters, Caveman, and so on. There are even diets based on your blood type, metabolic type, and astrological sign.

The problem is that the answers to our most fundamental questions change from one diet to the next. Different diet gurus tell us that fat, cholesterol, and carbohydrates are our enemies, even though each is a fundamental element of our biology. No one really says protein is the enemy (it is kind of like Switzerland), though some say you shouldn't have too much or your kidneys will fail. Can you ever get too much of Switzerland? Swiss cheese is full of protein, by the way. In Switzerland they use the metric system, and learning the metric system is probably the most useful thing you'll get out of counting grams of carbs or fat. Be careful though, statistics show that Americans had fewer heart attacks before they started trying to learn the metric system.[4]

While some nutrition gurus fight over which nutrients comprise the axis of evil, others focus on the miracle healing properties of supplements such as chromium, vanadium, herbal teas, and bitter melon. Such claims of natural remedies never go unanswered by the medical establishment who are always quick to remind us that supplements are unproven and may be harmful. Although the number of adverse reactions reported for most supplements is miniscule compared to that for prescription drugs, many doctors tell you to fear them as they dispense drugs like candy on Halloween.

Listening to diet gurus discuss their theories is like watching a presidential debate. Despite having completely opposite viewpoints, both sides sound unquestionably right. Each can cite a multitude of facts that support their unwavering ideology. Facts that don't support the party line are declared wrong, explained away, or simply ignored. Like political parties, dietary camps use the media to attack opposing theories and bombard the public with their ideologies. All this sugarcoating creates a great deal of confusion, which we are going to sort out with facts starting now.

Dietary clarity begins with an understanding of the four basic food groups. No, I don't mean milk, meat, vegetables, and bread (the old USDA "healthy" eating plan, for those of you fortunate enough to have not been subjected to it). I mean the four basic schools of dietary thought, or food theory camps. The four camps include the *Low Fat Fundamentalists*, captained by the famous Dr. Dean Ornish; the *Carbophobes* and their fearless leader Dr. Robert C. Atkins; the *Mods*, led by the omnipresent Dr. Walter Willett; and finally *The Establishment*, which is ruled by consensus committees and corporate sponsorship.

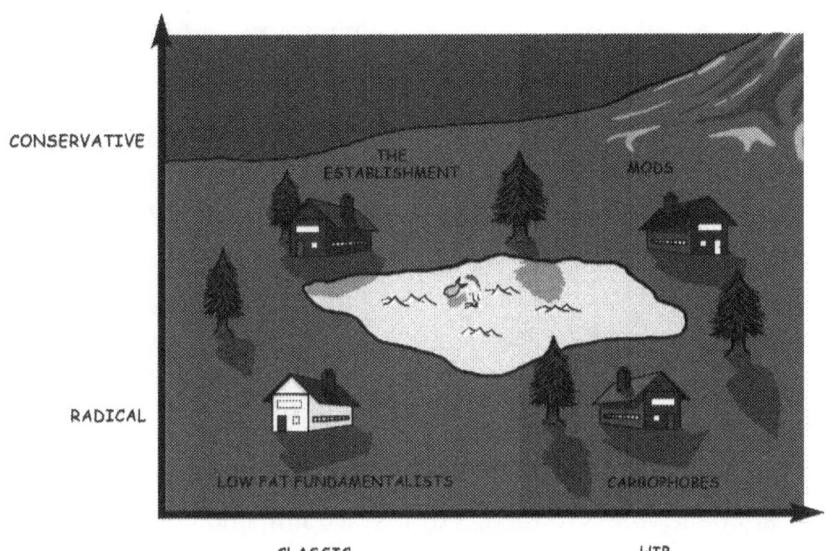

Figure 1: The Food Theory Campground

These four groups have positioned their campsites with respect to each other along the lines of two defining axes as illustrated in Figure 1, The Food Theory Campground. The horizontal "hipness" axis indicates how "in-style" the ideas reflected by the camp are, as evidenced by what's on the New York Times bestseller list and what everyone on the cast of *Friends* is doing. While the camps situated on the hip end base their ideas on the most recent research, those on the "classic" end seem to cling to the best research of the 60's, 70's, and early 80's, much in the same way classic rockers (like me) could care less about today's top 40. An important distinction between the east and west ends of this axis is "carb fear," which is new and cool, versus "fat fear," which is old and passé. While the *Mods* and *Carbophobes* are focused on incriminating carbohydrates, *The Establishment* and the *Low Fat Fundamentalists* maintain a steadfast preoccupation with vilifying dietary fat ... despite how 80's that makes them appear.

The vertical axis on our campground represents how conservative versus radical the ideology of a camp is. The camps on the upper side tend to be much more reserved and mainstream than their radical, fundamentalist, extremist neighbors to the south, who always seem to be starting some kind of revolution. Along this axis we find *The Establishment* and *Mods* aligned in the conservative region with *Low Fat Fundamentalists* and *Carbophobes* aligned in the radical zone. Camps on the southern end of the campground are hell bent on the belief that some nutrient is the evil enemy and that exorcising the demon from one's life is the only way to live long and stay healthy. Their less-orthodox counterparts to the north just recommend cutting back on the bad guy to correct some perceived imbalance. For example, while *The Establishment* recommends moderate consumption of oils, *Low Fat Fundamentalists* consider olive oil the juice of the devil. Whereas the *Mods* encourage consumption of fruits, vegetables, and whole grains, *Carbophobes* would sooner die than eat a slice of bread.

Now, while it's easy to poke fun at these groups (and we will) we should not lose sight of the fact that the work of everyone in the various camps has merit and is not to be discredited by simplistic labeling (hence we shall not use terms like "liberal" or "left of Ted Kennedy"). What we shall do is educate ourselves about the politics, dogma, and scientific evidence found in each camp, so that we can see through the sugarcoating and make informed decisions. This section will explore the competing ideologies on the campground and uncover the facts about diet.

2

The Carbophobes

Team Name:	Carbophobes
Team Captain:	Dr. Robert Atkins
Biggest Fear:	Carbs
Model Food:	T-Bone

Carbophobia, fear of the carbohydrate, is the diet rage of early 21st century America. What could be hipper than the diet used by Jennifer Lopez, Jennifer Anniston and Matthew Perry? The father of the modern carbophobic diet is the late Dr. Robert Atkins, honorary captain of the *Carbophobes*. Atkins is the diet where it's ok to eat the double bacon cheeseburger, just avoid the ketchup and throw out the bun. Chances are you or someone you know has tried the Atkins diet. You may even own one of the Atkins books; they have sold over fifteen million copies.

While the Atkins diet is primarily sold as a mechanism for weight loss, Atkins also claims that the diet can correct diabetes, heart disease, and high blood pressure because they are all consequences of carbohydrate overindulgence. The problem, according to Atkins, is that excessive consumption of refined carbohydrates (such as flour, sugar, and high-fructose corn syrup) causes a sharp rise in insulin and blood sugar levels, which results in storage of fat and the metabolic conditions related to obesity. Few would disagree with Atkins that refined carbohydrates should be limited. However, Atkins goes a step further into the radical zone by suggesting that severely limiting *all types* of carbohydrates is the key to reversing metabolic disorders like diabetes.

There is little doubt that the Atkins diet reduces insulin levels and burns excess fat. Losing extra weight is certainly one of the best things anyone with diabetes or other metabolic disorders can do to help themselves, but is strict limiting of carbohydrates necessarily the best and healthiest way to lose weight? According to Atkins, it is. His ultra low carb diet quickly exhausts the body's small supply of glycogen (stored glucose) forcing the body to enter a state called lipolysis, where it burns stored fat for energy. Because the body only enters lipolysis when deprived of carbohydrate, Atkins claims that his diet provides a "metabolic advantage." (Not to be confused with the *Atkins Advantage™* line of low carb chocolate bars, which offer luxurious chocolate taste with only 2 grams of "net carbs" per bar).

Thanks to this metabolic advantage, there is no need to count calories, just carbs. In *Dr. Atkins' New Diet Revolution*, Atkins admits, "It's true that gaining weight results from taking in more calories than you expend," but then says that "Atkins has repeatedly been proven to take off more fat than other programs when an equal number of calories is consumed." Does the physical law of conservation of energy bend to Atkins' metabolic advantage in some strange "quantum dietetics" kind of way? The evidence does not indicate so. Of the eight studies Atkins cites to back up his claim, only three used an equal number of calories in the groups studied, and none of these actually involved the Atkins diet.[5,6,7] Of the other five studies that didn't restrict calories, only two involved the Atkins diet.[8,9,10,11,12] One study compared the

Atkins diet to a starvation diet. As Newtonian physics would have it, subjects on the starvation diet lost more weight than those doing Atkins. Atkins argues that most of the weight lost by those fasting was lean body mass, and that those doing Atkins actually lost more fat. This may explain why starvation is not a good diet, but it doesn't support Atkins' theory that calories don't matter as long as you limit carbohydrates.

Calories do matter, but there is another side to the energy equation: energy *expenditure*. The amount of energy one expends, i.e., the number of calories ones burns, varies significantly depending on lean body mass, activity, and other factors (for example, starvation). Thus, if two diets with the same caloric intake result in different amounts of weight loss, it is likely due to a difference in energy expenditure, rather than a breakdown in the laws of Newtonian physics. Perhaps increased energy expenditure is the metabolic advantage Atkins refers to.

Atkins claims that a study performed by the Harvard Medical School in 2003 has provided evidence for this metabolic advantage. The study randomly assigned twenty-one participants to one of three separate diets:

1. a calorie-restricted low fat diet,
2. a calorie-restricted Atkins-style diet (same calorie amount as low fat diet), and
3. a calorie-restricted Atkins-style diet with 300 more calories per day than the other diets.

After twelve weeks, the results showed that both Atkins groups, even the one consuming 300 calories more, lost more weight than the low fat group.[13] However, the study report clearly states, "The difference between the diets was not statistically significant." This means that the observed differences were so small that they may just have been due to chance, like tossing a fair coin one hundred times and getting fifty-one heads versus forty-nine tails (for a detailed explanation of statistical significance, see Appendix A).

Nonetheless, Atkins cites this study as proof that "a low carb diet, with or without caloric restriction, produces greater weight loss than a low fat diet."[14] By citing a twelve-week study involving a handful of people that produced statistically insignificant results as proof of a metabolic advantage, Atkins is employing a common form of sugarcoating called *Glorification*. (Throughout this book I will identify common methods of sugarcoating using italicized names *Like This*.)

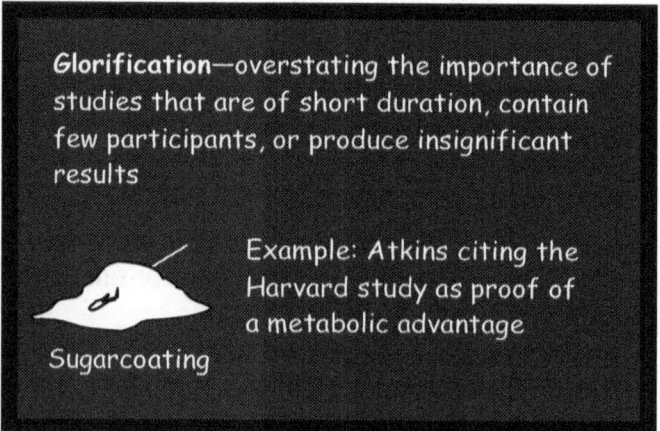

Chalkboard 2.1: Definition of Glorification

Atkins, like many nutrition theorists, liberally uses *Glorification* of small studies to create the impression that science has demonstrated the superiority of his diet.

Atkins' claim that the results of the Harvard study apply "with or without calorie restriction" employs another common form of sugarcoating called *Overgeneralization*: applying results to situations where they are inappropriate. By design, the Harvard study could not possibly support the "with or without calorie restriction" claim because all groups in the study were calorie restricted. Moreover, the Atkins diet isn't calorie restricted; you can eat as many calories as you want as long as you restrict carbohydrate intake. Once again, Atkins is citing a study that doesn't involve the Atkins diet. What would support the Atkins claim is a study in which participants were allowed to consume *unlimited* calories from Atkins bars, shakes, and low carb ice cream. The results of that study would be interesting.

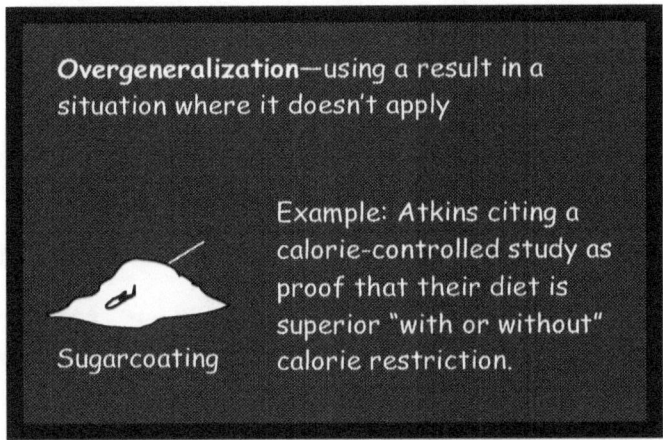

Overgeneralization—using a result in a situation where it doesn't apply

Example: Atkins citing a calorie-controlled study as proof that their diet is superior "with or without" calorie restriction.

Sugarcoating

Chalkboard 2.2: Definition of Overgeneralization

Atkins claims his diet is healthy because it promotes weight loss, which is one of the most effective means of preventing metabolic disorders. By this logic, any weight loss promoting diet (e.g., starvation) would be healthy. The question one must ask is whether the benefits of weight loss on the Atkins diet outweigh the potentially harmful effects. Atkins doesn't cite any studies that prove his diet improves outcomes for people with metabolic disorders, but there is no evidence that Atkins does any harm either. Still, critics have repeatedly stated the following concerns regarding Atkins and low carb diets:

1. High fat intake may be harmful to the cardiovascular system

2. High-protein intake may cause calcium loss and ultimately bone loss and speed the progression of diabetic kidney disease

3. Dieters may experience nutritional deficiency because they don't eat enough fruits and vegetables

Item 1 raises an important concern for us because heart disease is strongly associated with diabetes. However, there are no long-term studies showing a correlation between low carb diets and heart disease. This speculative claim is based on the theory that dietary fat raises total cholesterol and total cholesterol is a risk factor for heart disease. There are, however, many known risk factors for heart disease including the following:

- high blood levels of Low Density Lipoprotein (LDL) cholesterol

- low blood levels of High Density Lipoprotein (HDL) cholesterol

- high blood sugar

- high blood pressure

- high blood levels of triglycerides

- high blood levels of free fatty acids

It turns out that low carb diets actually improve many of these risk factors for heart disease. Studies involving low carb and low fat diets have been fairly consistent in showing that while low carb diets improve some risk factors (HDL cholesterol, triglycerides, and blood sugar) they worsen others (LDL cholesterol and free fatty acids) and that low fat diets have the opposite effects.[15,16,17,18,19,20,21,22,23] Thus, it appears the only way to improve all of the known risk factors is to simultaneously eat a low carb and low fat diet. We'll discuss the relationship between dietary fat, cholesterol, and heart disease in more detail in the next chapter on the *Low Fat Fundamentalists*.

Regarding item two, there is no clear evidence that high protein diets like Atkins produce calcium loss. Whereas calcium loss in the urine has been associated with diets containing greater than two to three times the U.S. Recommended Daily Allowance (RDA) for protein, other studies have shown that calcium retention was not reduced in a high meat diet versus low meat diet.[24,25,26] Factors other than dietary protein, for example, how often vegetables are consumed, may be involved. As for bone loss, a study that tracked over forty thousand women aged fifty-five to sixty-nine found that the risk of hip fracture, a common outcome related to bone loss, actually *decreased* as intake of animal protein increased.[27] With such conflicting evidence, it is speculative to link high protein diets to bone loss. Moreover, there is no evidence that, for the vast majority of diabetics who do not already have diabetic kidney disease, eating more protein and fewer carbohydrates will increase the risk of kidney damage. On the contrary, keeping blood sugars down by controlling carbohydrates can prevent kidney disease and other complications from occurring in the first place. According to Dr. Richard K. Bernstein, "High levels of dietary protein do not cause kidney disease in diabetics or anyone else." His best selling book, *Dr. Bernstein's Diabetes Solution,* gives an excellent, evidence-based explanation of how high blood sugar, not dietary protein, leads to kidney disease.

Item three regarding nutritional deficiency is perhaps the only valid health concern with the Atkins diet. In his book, Dr. Atkins sings the praises of vegetables, especially the leafy green, low carb, ones. However, his diet prohibits high carb vegetables (e.g. peas, carrots, and corn) and allows only one cup of "cooking" vegetables (e.g. broccoli, spinach, and cauliflower) plus two cups of "salad" vegetables (e.g. celery, lettuce, and cucumbers) per day. Atkins admits that this regimen may result in vitamin and mineral deficiency and recommends a multivitamin supplement during the initial phase of his diet. Subsequent phases of the diet allow increased but still limited amounts of vegetables and the introduction of small amounts of nuts and berries. However, in all phases carbs are strictly controlled. While the later phases of Atkins may appear on paper to be nutritionally sound, one has to wonder how many Atkins dieters are following these guidelines. How many are following the "maintenance" phase, eating spinach and raspberries and drinking four ounces of tomato juice as opposed to eating Atkins Advantage™ bars and drinking Atkins shakes? While it is *theoretically possible* to get adequate nutrition on Atkins, the *reality* is that it isn't likely to happen on a diet of low carb shakes, "nutrition" bars, and sugar-free products. Consuming these products is equivalent to eating their empty calorie counterparts with a low-dose vitamin pill, with one difference: replacement of sugar with sugar alcohols to lower the so-called "net carb" count.

Sugar alcohols (e.g., maltitol, lacitol, and sorbitol) are starches that contain calories. While U.S. law requires that they be reported as carbohydrates and included in calorie counts on food labels, Atkins gets around this by displaying the "net carbs" designation prominently on product wrappers. The small print on the back of the label explains that fiber and sugar alcohols have a "negligible" effect on blood sugar and thus you can ignore them. This allows an Atkins chocolate bar containing 24 grams of carbs to be advertised as having only 3 grams of net carbs. By creating the illusion that the candy bar is a healthy, guilt-free snack, the net carbs designation employs a classic form of sugarcoating known as *Guiltabsolution*.

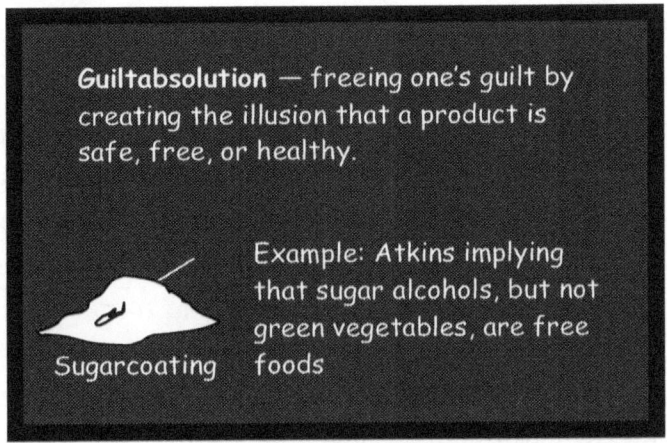

Guiltabsolution — freeing one's guilt by creating the illusion that a product is safe, free, or healthy.

Example: Atkins implying that sugar alcohols, but not green vegetables, are free foods

Sugarcoating

Chalkboard 2.3: Definition of Guiltabsolution

When it comes to sugar alcohol carbs, Atkins is remarkably lenient. Most sugar alcohols affect blood sugar as much as green vegetables, nuts, and seeds, which are strictly limited on the Atkins diet. Maltitol, which has been used in Atkins products, has a greater impact on blood sugar than these foods, yet there is no limit on the intake of maltitol or any other sugar alcohols. Although the first edition of *Dr. Atkins' New Diet Revolution* clearly stated: "Sweeteners such as sorbitol, mannitol and other hexitols are not allowed," that phrase was removed in the 2002 edition. [28]

Nonetheless, there is one compelling benefit of the low carb diet for diabetics: *eating fewer carbs means lower blood sugar.* Indeed, there is an abundance of evidence that low carb diets result in lower fasting and post-meal blood sugars as well as a reduction in HbA1c. [29,30,31,32,33,34,35] Whether you are overweight or not, the low carb diet can reduce spikes in your blood glucose. According to

Dr. Bernstein, "Big inputs make big mistakes; small inputs make small mistakes." Bernstein explains how the same amount of uncertainty in estimating carb content can result in a 150 mg/dl swing in blood sugar for a bowl of pasta but only a 20 mg/dl change for a low carb salad.[36] The difference can be even larger if you are taking insulin, which adds more variability to the equation.

Despite the sugarcoating coming from the *Carbophobes*, it appears that low carb diets can provide health benefits, especially for diabetics. Bear in mind that no study has ever shown that a diet of Atkins Advantage™ bars and shakes will make you lose weight or improve your HbA1c levels. Those improvements came on tightly controlled diets that involved replacing refined carbohydrates with healthy fats and protein, not sugar alcohols. Success in low carb dieting comes only with a deep appreciation for Dr. Atkins' often forgotten message to get your carbohydrates from nutrient rich, fibrous vegetables. If you follow this advice and stay away from low carb junk food then eating a little beef probably won't give you a heart attack. There are some however, who would strongly disagree with this. Dr. Dean Ornish and his disciples, the *Low Fat Fundamentalists*, are the subjects of our next chapter.

3

The Low Fat Fundamentalists

Team Name: Low Fat Fundamentalists
Team Captain: Dr. Dean Ornish
Biggest Fear: Fat
Model Food: Rice Cake

The real reason people lose weight on Atkins-style diets, say the *Low Fat Fundamentalists*, is because when they stop eating carbohydrates they also reduce their intake of fats as well—the fat in pasta sauces, the cream cheese on a bagel. A gram of fat has twice as many calories as a gram of carbohydrates, so if you restrict fat you can eat more and lose weight. Fat, whether it comes from a vegetable or animal, is the evil nutrient and avoiding it will prevent heart disease and make us all live longer. This is the Gospel according to Dr. Dean Ornish, captain of the *Low Fat Fundamentalists*.

Heart disease is an important concern for diabetics because we are at increased risk of getting it. If there is a diet that can reduce our risk of heart disease, we should, of course, follow it. But is a low fat diet really a heart healthy diet?

Dr. Ornish has demonstrated that heart disease can be reversed using his lifestyle intervention program, which includes an ultra low fat vegetarian diet, daily exercise, weight loss, meditation, and group therapy. The Ornish program was associated with a reversal of coronary blockage when compared to a control group who received "usual care." Twenty-three of twenty-eight patients following the program exhibited some reversal of their coronary blockages.[37] The power of lifestyle intervention to reverse heart disease echoes the results of similar large-scale studies showing how lifestyle interventions can halt the progression of diabetes.[38,39,40]

Ornish's lifestyle intervention program is rigorous to say the least. It calls for a vegetarian diet that is ultra low in salt, sugar, and fat (the three staples of the American diet), and allows no cholesterol, meat, fish, coffee, or anything else you might call "fun." Participants in Ornish's program are given a customized exercise plan that in the first year averages one hour per day, five days a week. They meditate for an hour and a half every day of the week and participate in four-hour group therapy sessions twice a week. With all these major lifestyle changes, it's no surprise that the study participants lost an average of twenty-four pounds in the first year.[41]

Are you ready to sign up? Before committing to five major lifestyle changes at once, you might like to know which parts of this program actually made a difference and which didn't. If diet turned out to be important, you may want to know specifically which parts of the diet mattered before you go trading in cheesecake for rice cakes. Knowing what specific changes work might save you a lot of time and avoid needless self-deprivation.

The problem is, as Ornish admits, "We don't know the relative contribution of each component of the program. That is, we can't say how much of the improvement was due to the changes in diet, how much was from the stress management techniques, how much was due to the group support and so on."[42] All we know is that when all of them are done together good things happen. It may well be that if you follow an Atkins diet, exercise, meditate, and attend group therapy then you can also reverse heart disease. Maybe just the exercise and meditation will do the trick. The point is, *we don't know*. Nonetheless, Ornish cites this study as evidence that his low fat, vegetarian diet works to reverse heart disease.

Lumping a number of factors together so that the contribution of each is not clear and then attributing success to a single factor is a method of sugarcoating called *Obfuscation*.

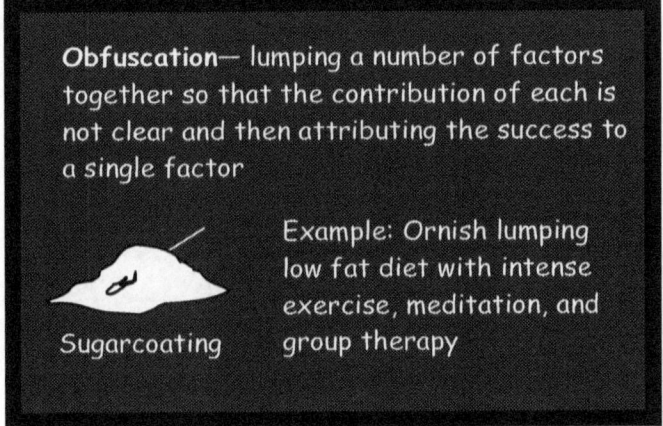

Obfuscation— lumping a number of factors together so that the contribution of each is not clear and then attributing the success to a single factor

Example: Ornish lumping low fat diet with intense exercise, meditation, and group therapy

Sugarcoating

Chalkboard 3.1: Definition of Obfuscation

While there is some evidence of benefit from each of the components of Ornish's program, the ultra low fat diet is scientifically on the shakiest ground. The argument goes like this: eating fat makes you fatter because every gram of fat contains nine calories versus only four for carbohydrates. That sounds simple enough. In fact, it's too simplistic to be of any use to us. Looking a little closer we find that, whereas carbohydrates are used *exclusively* for energy, protein and fat are used for *partially* for energy but also to build cells and hormones. Moreover, when proteins and fats reach the stomach and again when they reach the small intestine, "full" signals are sent to the brain to suppress hunger. With carbohydrates, however, the full signal comes later. Thus it is easier to overeat carbohydrates (e.g. rice cakes) than fat/protein foods (e.g. eggs). When people try to cut the fat out of their diets they often just make up the calories in carbohydrates. Perhaps the most damning evidence against the "calorie per gram" theory comes from the numerous studies in which people have lost more weight on low carb diets than low fat ones.[43,44,45,46,47,48,49]

By focusing solely on calories per gram and ignoring other important factors involved in digestion, the *Low Fat Fundamentalists* are employing a common form of sugarcoating called *Ignorisolation*.

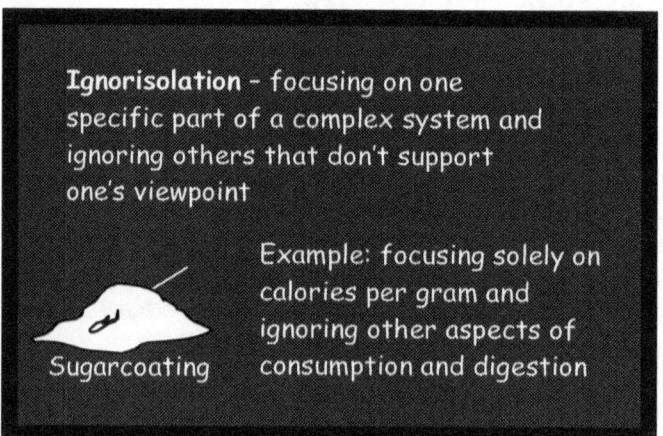

Chalkboard 3.2: Definition of Ignorisolation

Surely the *Low Fat Fundamentalists* are aware that dietary fat is needed for healthy skin, vitamin absorption, building cell membranes, strengthening the immune system, metabolizing cholesterol, and maintaining your brain, which, incidentally, is mostly composed of fat. The standard *Low Fat Fundamentalist* response to these biological facts is found in the book, *Dr. Dean*

Ornish's Program For Reversing Heart Disease. Whereas Ornish acknowledges that there are essential fats that your body can only get through diet, he immediately adds, "The average person needs to consume less than fourteen grams of fat to meet the daily requirements."[50]

Perhaps Ornish is using the words "average person" here to mean "average woman" because the dietary reference intake (DRI) for the two strictly essential fatty acids, linoleic acid and alpha linolenic acid, for women is about fourteen grams but not for adult men. The DRI for males aged nineteen to fifty is about nineteen grams. The number is even higher if we include the vital but only conditionally essential fatty acids eicosapentaenoic acid (EPA) and docosahexaenoic acid (DHA).

Whereas it is *theoretically possible* to consume the dietary reference intakes without any other fat by taking a perfectly balanced, purely extracted supplement, the *reality* is that food happens to contain other types of fat. Getting the dietary reference intakes of essential fatty acids from diet requires eating far more than just the number of grams of fat stated in the DRI for two essential fatty acids. Ornish's statement employs *Ignorisolation*, by focusing on the reference intakes of two specific fatty acids and ignoring the *reality* of how one gets these essential fats from diet. Does the Ornish Reversal Diet allow consumption of fish oil supplements, canola oil, or anything with a high enough concentration of essential fatty acids to come anywhere near his theoretical goal? No.[51] However, in a reversal of his reversal diet, Ornish in 1994 began recommending fish oil supplements.[52]

The Ornish diet strictly forbids olive oil, which is generally accepted as one of the most heart healthy substances on the planet. When countries around the globe were compared, the lowest incidence of heart disease was found in the neighboring regions of Greece, Crete, and southern Italy, where the diet, commonly called the Mediterranean Diet, consists of forty percent fat and plenty of olive oil.[53] Numerous studies have since shown the Mediterranean diet to be associated with a reduced rate of death from heart disease, cancer, and all causes.[54,55,56] Olive oil is made up of approximately seventy percent monounsaturated fat, which reduces most risk factors for heart disease.[57] However, Ornish and the *Low Fat Fundamentalists* maintain that olive oil should be avoided because it contains some amount of saturated fat, and will thus raise cholesterol and increase risk for heart disease. Once again the *Low Fat Fundamentalists* are employing *Ignorisolation* by focusing on the negative effects of one type of fat and ignoring the positive effects of the other.

According to Ornish, dietary fat is what makes you fat so you can and should eat plenty of carbohydrates, as long as they are the "complex" kind. Ornish knows that the body converts excess carbohydrates into fat and cholesterol, so his diet is low in what he calls "simple" carbohydrates.

What exactly are "complex" and "simple" carbohydrates anyway? Does one have some kind of deep, dark, mysterious, psychologically distraught personality while the other is just really down to earth? Actually, the complex/simple terminology is a relic of a very old, yet still pervasive dietary theory. The theory suggests that since complex carbohydrates (e.g. those found in pasta) are made up of large molecules containing long chains of glucose, they are more slowly digested and absorbed than the tiny molecules found in simple carbohydrates (e.g. sugar). Therefore simple carbohydrates should have a faster and greater effect on blood sugar.

It turns out that this theory is wrong. Standardized measurements performed on hundreds of subjects and over seven hundred different kinds of carbohydrate foods have shown that some "complex" carbohydrates, like rice and corn flakes, raise blood sugar more than "simple" carbohydrates like jellybeans and Coca-Cola.[58] Some complex carbohydrates are so quickly absorbed that they raise blood levels of glucose and triglycerides (fat), increase the risk of diabetes and heart disease, and, as the old saying about Chinese food goes, make you hungry again an hour later.[59,60,61]

Saying "complex carbohydrate" is like saying "groovy," it identifies you as coming from way out on the classic end of the campground. Even the American Diabetes Association, which is firmly planted in "Classicland," recommends avoiding such terms.[62]

By sticking with an outdated complex carbohydrate theory, Ornish effectively equates rice cakes, which raise blood glucose faster than chocolate bars, with broccoli. Depending on which type of complex carbohydrate you eat freely on the Ornish diet you will either stay trim and healthy or become overweight and unhealthy. Such *Obfuscation* is a recurring problem in Ornish's program; things like exercise and stress reduction are lumped in with unproven ideas like his ultra low fat, complex carbohydrate diet. It's not clear what is really helping, what isn't, and what may be having a negative effect.

Nonetheless, there persists the belief that there is a large body of scientific evidence supporting the linkage between dietary fat and heart disease. There isn't. There is, however, a long history of clinical trials that failed to prove this theory, called the diet-heart hypothesis.

The diet-heart hypothesis was first put forth in the 1950's by biochemist Ancel Keys. When Keys was born in 1904, infectious diseases were the leading cause of death in the United States and coronary heart disease (CHD) was relatively rare.[63] Throughout Keys' lifetime the incidence of coronary heart disease steadily increased and, by the 1950's, had become the leading cause of death in the United States. Keys began looking around the world to discover why the incidence of coronary heart disease was so much higher in the United States than other countries. He quickly arrived at the answer: high-fat food. He supported his theory with a diagram (similar to that shown in chalkboard 3.3) showing a "clear" correlation between the total intake of fat and coronary heart disease in six countries.

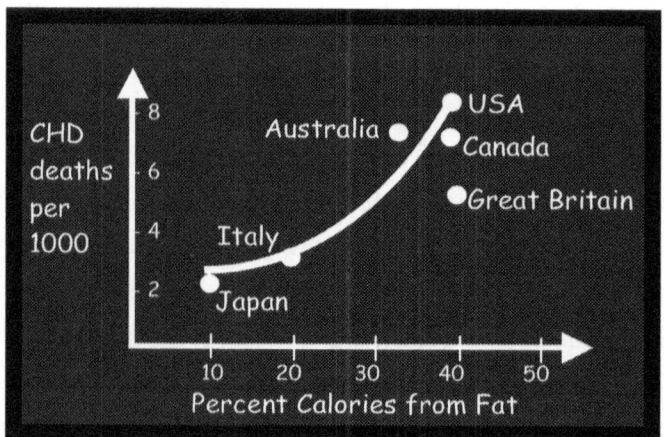

Chalkboard 3.3: Fat consumption versus coronary heart disease (CHD) in six countries (data from Keys[64])

The data points for Keys' figure were computed based on the amount of fat available for consumption in each country (not the actual amounts eaten by people) and the cause of death written on death certificates. Whether or not these metrics are useful enough to prove the point is of no consequence because the graph was produced using a form of sugarcoating called *Selective Omission.*

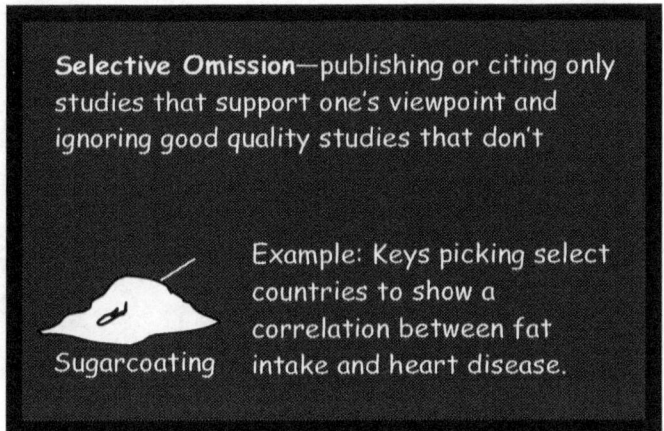

Chalkboard 3.4: Definition of Selective Omission

As Dr. Uffe Ravnskov points out in *The Cholesterol Myths,* fat production and death certificate data was available from twenty-two countries at the time Keys performed this study.[65] When all twenty-two countries are plotted, the correlation disappears.[66] Had Keys chosen, for example, the countries of Chile, Israel, Austria, France, Holland, and Sweden for his study, he could have shown that eating more fat is correlated with a *lower* incidence of death from coronary heart disease, as illustrated in Chalkboard 3.5.

Although some criticized Keys' theory, it became the foundation of heart disease prevention, and the diet-heart hypothesis, version 1.0, was born. Whereas contradictory evidence, accumulated over the course of half a century, has forced significant modification of the original theory (Figures 3.6 and 3.8), public awareness has been anchored to the over-simplified, erroneous message of version 1.0, that dietary fat causes heart disease. This is due, in no small part, to sugarcoating, as we shall now see.

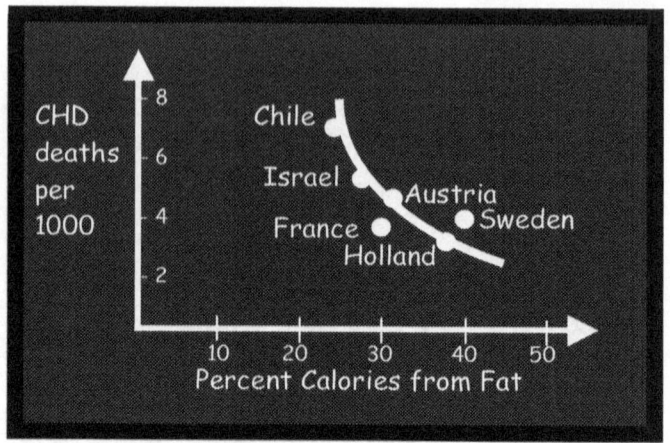

Chalkboard 3.5: Fat consumption versus coronary heart disease (CHD) in six countries (data from Yerushalmy and Hilleboe[67])

Once the diet-heart hypothesis was put forth, several studies investigating the relationship between dietary fat and heart disease ensued. One of the first was Ancel Keys' landmark Seven Countries Study, which examined the lifestyles and incidence of coronary heart disease in eighteen populations in seven countries.[68,69] The Seven Countries Study showed Keys' theory was wrong; the populations that had the lowest incidence of coronary heart disease consumed a very high fat, Mediterranean diet. Thus Keys revised the diet-heart hypothesis to state that:

Consumption of animal fat increased risk for CHD, and eating more vegetable fat decreased it.

The Seven Countries Study also linked blood cholesterol to heart disease. Keys demonstrated a correlation between cholesterol levels and heart disease, but only when grouping populations by country (*Obfuscation*). Keys did not explain why populations within a country having similar cholesterol levels had such widely varying rates of heart disease. This was a problem that would beset many dietary fat and cholesterol studies to come.

A positive correlation between cholesterol levels and death from coronary heart disease was found in the Framingham Heart Study, which monitored over five thousand people in the town of Framingham, Massachusetts for several years.[70,71] However, this result was observed only in a certain age group. The relationship weakened and even reversed with increasing age suggesting that higher cholesterol levels were actually *heart-protective* for older people. Digging deeper, Framingham researchers had found that, in the elderly, heart disease was more strongly correlated with a specific type of cholesterol (LDL), and inversely correlated with another type (HDL).[72] Subsequently, LDL cholesterol was labeled "bad," HDL cholesterol "good," and the diet-heart hypothesis metamorphosized, yet again, into a rather contorted form:

Bad cholesterol causes CHD and good cholesterol prevents it. Animal fats raise total cholesterol, which includes bad cholesterol, so animal fats must cause CHD

This version of the theory leads one to wonder about the so-called *good* cholesterol that animal fats also raise. Since animal fats improve the ratio of good to bad cholesterol, wouldn't they be healthy according to this theory? This sort of inquiry has been systematically drowned out by *Ignorisolation* sugarcoating, ignoring any risk factor other than LDL cholesterol to make dietary fat the villain.

The evolution of the diet-heart hypothesis from 1950 through 1970 is shown in Chalkboard 3.6 below.

Diet-Heart Hypothesis (1950-1970)

~~Dietary fat causes CHD~~

Animal fat causes CHD, ~~but vegetable fat prevents~~ CHD

~~Animal fat raises~~ cholesterol, which causes CHD

Bad LDL cholesterol causes CHD, though good HDL prevents it. Animal fat raises total cholesterol, which includes LDL so animal fat must cause CHD

Chalkboard 3.6: The Diet-Heart Hypothesis (1950-1970)

The Framingham study provided no evidence that those who ate less fat lived longer or had fewer heart attacks. Ironically, the participants who consumed more fat and cholesterol actually had lower blood cholesterol. The reason, according to study director, Dr. William Castelli, is that "the people who ate the most cholesterol, ate the most saturated fat, ate the most calories, weighed the least and were the most physically active."[73] (Could this be Atkins' metabolic advantage?) Whatever the explanation, the results from Framingham should have been enough to discard the diet-heart hypothesis in 1970. Three other government funded studies conducted around the same time in Honolulu, Chicago, and Puerto Rico similarly failed to substantiate the diet-heart hypothesis.[74] In fact, no large-scale study has ever shown that eating less fat reduces risk of heart disease. The only thing reproducible and consistent about early diet-heart studies is their *failure* to show dietary fat affecting any outcomes.

Nonetheless, the National Heart, Lung, and Blood Institute (NHLBI) continued pouring money into studies investigating the link between saturated fat, cholesterol, and heart disease. One such study, the Multiple Risk Factor Intervention Trial (MRFIT) involved 12,866 high-risk men, aged thirty-five to fifty-seven, who were selectively chosen from a pool of 360,000 candidates. Since diet alone was unlikely to produce much difference in outcome, the study designers combined a low fat diet with advice to exercise, quit smoking, and lose weight (*Obfuscation*, Ornish style). Despite these efforts the study still did not produce any statistically significant differences in deaths from heart disease or overall mortality between groups.[75] However, as Dr. Ravenskov noted, heart disease mortality rates in MRFIT were about 50% lower in those who quit smoking, whether in the treatment group or not.[76,77] These data suggest that some lifestyle changes (e.g. quitting smoking) can help prevent heart disease, but eating a low fat diet is not among them.

Henceforth came a new and creative way for establishing a support for the diet-heart hypothesis: it would be logically "deduced" using results from two independent lines of research:

1. research showing that eating a specific type of fat raised total cholesterol levels

2. proof that lowering total cholesterol prevented heart attacks.

Combining the two with a good dose of sugarcoating would produce the desired conclusion: *low fat diets prevent heart attacks*.

Along the first line, experiments showed that most saturated fats raise levels of both LDL and HDL cholesterol.[78] However, it was also found that stearic acid, a saturated fatty acid commonly found in red meat and butter, has no effect on any type of cholesterol.[79] Inconsistencies like this would not hinder the diet-heart hypothesis; they would ultimately be buried in *Obfuscation* and *Overgeneralization*. The message, *eating fat raises cholesterol and is thus bad for you,* would not distinguish among specific types of fat, specific types of cholesterol, or the specific type of patients to which the findings applied.

It was a very specific finding, in fact, that was used to establish the second line of support for the diet-heart hypothesis. The goal of the NHLBI's multi-million dollar Lipids Research Clinics (LRC) trial was to show that lowering cholesterol with medication could reduce the incidence of CHD. To provide the best chance to produce meaningful results, the study's designers selected only middle-aged men whose cholesterol levels exceeded those of ninety-five percent of Americans for participation (*Selective Omission*). Half were given a cholesterol-lowering drug and the other half a placebo. After seven years, the drug-taking group lowered their total cholesterol more than the placebo group (8.5 percent, or a drop of forty points vs. thirty-seven points) and those on drugs experienced fewer heart attacks than those in the placebo group (7.0 percent versus 8.6 percent).[80] Whether these small differences were the result of chance was the subject of much debate.[81,82] In the six years following the publication of these results, chance reversed its course with more new heart attacks occurring in the drug group than in the placebo group.[83] After thirteen years, the difference in heart disease between the drug and placebo groups stood at a mere 0.9 percent.

Nonetheless, the six-year LRC results led to the oft-repeated mantra "For each one percent reduction in cholesterol, we can expect a two percent reduction in CHD events." Does this mean that a fifty percent reduction in cholesterol results in a one hundred percent reduction in heart disease? What about a sixty percent reduction? Would you get twenty bonus points to apply to your next lifetime? No. This is a form of sugarcoating called *Mislinearization.*

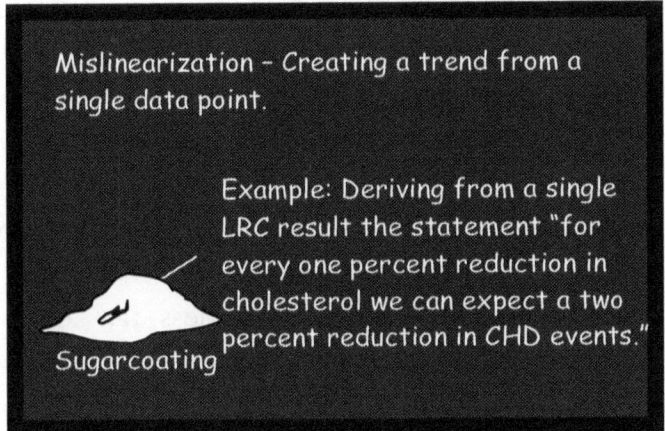

Mislinearization – Creating a trend from a single data point.

Example: Deriving from a single LRC result the statement "for every one percent reduction in cholesterol we can expect a two percent reduction in CHD events."

Sugarcoating

Chalkboard 3.7: Definition of Mislinearization

The statement is derived from just one data point, but implies there is a linear trend (which, according to Euclid, requires at least two points). Worse, it ignores a second key data point, the six-year follow-up study, which shows an opposite trend and calls into question the statistical significance of the entire study (*Selective Omission*). At best, the LRC results were highly specific: for middle-aged men with very high cholesterol, taking cholesterol-lowering medication for thirteen years reduced their chances of having a heart attack from fifteen percent to fourteen percent.

Let's use this fact to create another example of *Mislinearization*. Since, over the course of thirteen years, the pharmaceutical industry earns over a hundred billion dollars from the sales of cholesterol-lowering medication, the LRC results show that:

For every billion dollars in revenue from cholesterol-lowering medication we can expect a one one-hundredth of one percent improvement in preventing heart attacks.

The most ironic thing about the LRC trial is that, although diet was not a variable in the study, the trial was miraculously hailed as the long-awaited proof of the diet-heart hypothesis. The voices of reason that tried to point out the obvious flaws in this argument were drowned out by a massive media campaign, which included a frowning face on a plate of bacon and eggs on the cover of Time magazine. Almost overnight low fat products began to flood the market. Despite a plethora of contrary evidence, the over-simplified, over-generalized message, "eat less fat, lower your cholesterol, and prevent heart attacks," became the mantra for a generation.

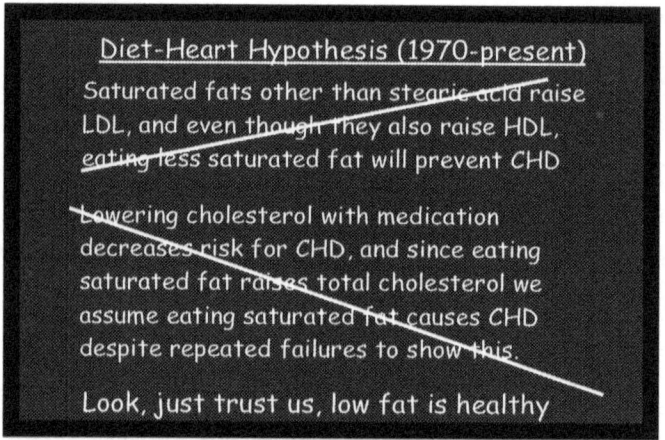

Chalkboard 3.8: The Diet-Heart Hypothesis (1970-present)

That generation appears to be ending as the evidence against the diet-heart hypothesis continues to mount. In February 2006 the results from the Women's Health Initiative Randomized Controlled Dietary Modification Trial were published. After following 48,835 women for eight years, the study found no difference in the rates of heart attack, stroke, breast cancer, and colon cancer between those on a low fat diet and those on a high fat diet.[84,85,86]

The clerics of low fat fundamentalism are well aware of the evidence that contradicts their dogmatic claims. They don't deny that high-carbohydrate diets raise triglycerides and decrease (good) HDL cholesterol—both risk factors for heart disease.[87,88] However, Dr. Ornish rationalizes that when you are eating a low fat, low cholesterol diet you have less need for HDL. He says, "We need to move beyond simplistic notions that anything that raises HDL-C is beneficial and anything that lowers HDL-C is harmful."[89] Ironically, the *Low Fat Fundamentalist* ideology hinges on the simplistic notion that anything that lowers LDL-C is beneficial and anything that raises LDL-C is harmful.

Indeed, we do need to move beyond simplistic notions related to fat and cholesterol, especially those coming from fundamentalists like Ornish and being reinforced by the government, health organizations, medical professionals, and the mass media. How and why *The Establishment* sugarcoats dietary advice is the subject of the next chapter.

4

The Establishment

Team Name: The Establishment
Team Captain: Committee and corporate sponsors
Biggest Fear: Fat, Loss of corporate sponsorship
Model Food: Sponsors' products

The Establishment is undoubtedly the dominant camp in dietary theory. Made up of doctors, nurses, educators, dieticians, other health care professionals, researchers, journalists, universities, government organizations, consumer advocacy groups, non-profit health organizations, and funded by numerous food and drug companies, *The Establishment* is everywhere. Its message to eat less fat and cholesterol has been the official word on diet for decades now, appearing everywhere from journals to pamphlets to popular magazines.

The Establishment's messages are promulgated by large non-profit organizations such as the American Diabetes Association (ADA), American Heart Association (AHA), and American Dietetic Association (another ADA), as well as government organizations such as the National Heart, Lung, and Blood Institute (NHLBI), National Cholesterol Education Program (NCEP) and United States Department of Agriculture (USDA). Whereas these organizations are often treated like infallible sources of enlightened wisdom, they all have interests that conflict with giving unbiased dietary advice. They may exist to promote the agricultural industry (like the USDA), rely heavily on corporate sponsorship (like the ADA and AHA), or simply have committees stacked with individuals with known financial ties to food industries creating a conflict of interest (like the NCEP and USDA).

In July of 2004 NCEP unveiled its new guidelines for target cholesterol levels, which, as it turned out, made millions of new people eligible for cholesterol-lowering drugs. Although this wasn't originally disclosed, eight of the nine members of the NCEP panel creating the guidelines had received research grants, speaking honoraria, or consulting fees from manufacturers of cholesterol-lowering drugs.[90] In 2000, a federal court ruled that the USDA violated federal laws by appointing panel members with known financial ties to food industries to the Dietary Guidelines Advisory Committee, the committee responsible for advising the nation on diet through its *Dietary Guidelines for Americans* and the Food Guide Pyramid.[91]

The USDA Dietary Guidelines reflect the organization's dual goals of giving the public nutritional advice and promoting U.S. agriculture. When the USDA was created in 1862, these goals were mostly in line with each other. However, the twentieth century saw the leading causes of death in the United States change from infectious diseases such as pneumonia/influenza and tuberculosis to chronic diseases such as heart disease, cancer, and stroke.[92] The new advice—that Americans should eat less and lose weight—has come in conflict with the goal of promoting the consumption of American-made agricultural products such as grain and dairy.

This conflict manifests itself in the unrealistically small portion sizes defined in the USDA's pyramid and dietary guidelines. There is a wide disparity between USDA servings and the servings Americans typically put on their plates or are served in restaurants. Industry pressure, which led to the retraction of the first Food Guide Pyramid in 1991, has resulted in a pyramid where portion sizes are so small that the number of allowable or recommended portions is unrealistically high. When the second, more industry-friendly version of the pyramid was introduced in 1992, it recommended six to eleven servings of grains per day. Most people don't realize that a large muffin can meet this recommendation.

By using deceptively small portions to encourage greater consumption, the Food Guide Pyramid exemplifies a form of sugarcoating called *Minification*. This has made the pyramid a useful marketing tool for American made grain products. This is why depictions of it frequently appear on the labels of pasta, cereal, bread, and other foods that benefit from the USDA's implicit endorsement. It is not surprising that total food consumption and obesity have risen since the introduction of the Food Guide Pyramid.

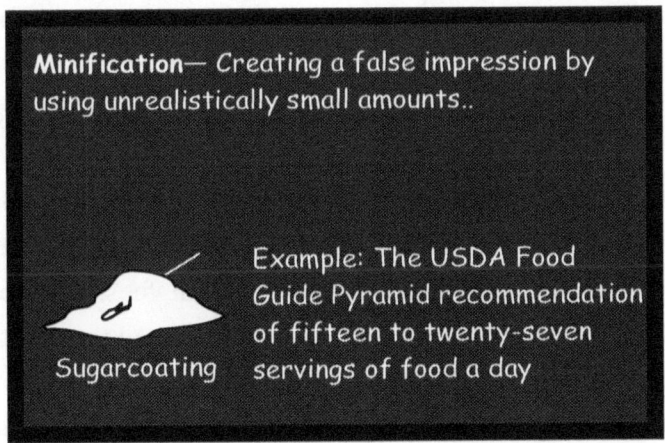

Minification— Creating a false impression by using unrealistically small amounts..

Example: The USDA Food Guide Pyramid recommendation of fifteen to twenty-seven servings of food a day

Sugarcoating

Chalkboard 4.1: Definition of Minification

How industry pressure influences the USDA Advisory Committee guidelines has been thoroughly documented by nutritionist and former member of the Advisory Committee, Marion Nestle.[93] According to Nestle, one of the main reasons food industry lobbyists work so hard to influence the nutritional recommendations is that subtle changes in perception make large differences in product sales. This is why food companies spend millions of dollars on advertising just to create the perception that Coca-Cola® is better than Pepsi® or low fat cookies are healthier than regular ones.

In November of 1991 CBS aired a *60 Minutes* segment on the "French Paradox" that affirmed the health benefits of red wine. After the segment, sales of red wine increased nearly 45% and shortages caused a sharp rise in the prices of Californian wines. The audience for *60 Minutes* is large, but nutritional advice from the U.S. government has a much broader reach. Accordingly, food industry lobbyists work to make sure the government doesn't hinder the sales of their products. Corporations are very sensitive to any "eat less" or "drink less" messages related to their products, and will protest vehemently and even litigate against the slightest insinuation that people should consume less of their product.

In one of the most publicized cases, Oprah Winfrey and one of her guests were sued by Texas cattlemen for a 1996 show that, according to the cattlemen, falsely and maliciously condemned U.S. beef and resulted in a beef market crash. Oprah was found innocent, but spent a million dollars in legal fees. This price tag makes the threat of litigation a very real consideration for journalists making statements that might in any way affect sales of some food product. In 2004 it was reported that the Florida Citrus Growers, upset over loss of sales due to low carb dieting, were considering litigation against authors of low carb books such as

The South Beach Diet.[94]

No one, including the World Health Organization (WHO), is immune. In the days leading up to the release of the 2003 *The World Health Organization Expert Report on Diet*, which included explicit recommendations to limit sugar, the U.S. Sugar Association threatened to "exercise every avenue available to expose the dubious nature" of the expert report. Their lobbyists had congressmen urging the U.S. Secretary of Health, Tommy Thompson, to cut off the U.S. funding of the WHO unless the WHO retracted its report.[95] The U.S. Department of Health and Human Services wrote to the WHO harshly criticizing their proposition that heavy marketing of high-sugar products and fast foods is related to obesity.[96]

The U.S. sugar industry has been rather successful in its efforts to prevent the U.S. government from issuing recommendations against its product. The government-mandated Nutrition Facts panel contains recommended daily values for all listed nutrients with one notable omission: sugar. Whereas the government has specified, down to the percentage point, how much saturated fat, polyunsaturated fat, and monounsaturated fat Americans should consume, it makes only vague comments about sugar. Marion Nestle described the situation surrounding the 2000 update to the USDA guideline for sugar as follows:

> *Last September, the draft guideline said: "Go easy on beverages and foods high in added sugars." Complaints from the sugar industry led to the February draft, "Choose beverages and foods that limit our intake of sugars," and eventually to the summit version: "Choose beverages and foods to moderate your intake of sugars."* [97]

Manufacturers of sugar-based products can improve their

public image by sponsoring non-profit organizations that provide influential dietary recommendations. Their sponsorship dollars are a major source of funding for the non-profits and appear to earn them the right of censorship of any health messages these groups put out.

Censorship by way of sponsorship, or *Spensorship*, is a form of sugarcoating that constrains dietary advice coming from information authorities such as the American Diabetes Association. Among the numerous food companies and pharmaceutical companies that generously sponsor the ADA (Table 4.1) you will find companies such as General Mills, Murray Sugar Free Cookies, Voortman Cookies, Hershey, Nestle, and Coca-Cola. The ADA does not publish statements like "sugar-free cookies are high in refined carbohydrates" or "soft drinks are full of sugar." They do, however, have a campaign for dispelling the myth that sugar causes diabetes, as if confusion on this matter were some kind of major public health issue. It isn't, but the public's perceptions about sugar are extremely important to ADA sponsors.

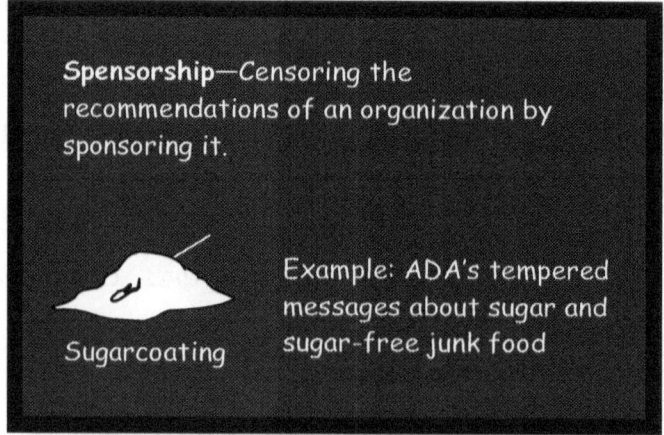

Chalkboard 4.2: Definition of Spensorship

Sponsorship virtually guarantees that the nutritional advice you get from non-profit organizations will not be displeasing to sponsors and will not change, even in light of new important developments that are accepted by scientists working within these very organizations. In 2002 the ADA published an extensive survey of dietary research for diabetics, *Evidence-Based Nutrition Principles and Recommendations for the Treatment and Prevention of Diabetes and Related Complications.*[98] The normative text of this fifty-page report acknowledges current research showing that some fats are heart-healthy, and that high carbohydrate diets can negatively affect blood glucose, insulin, triglycerides, and HDL cholesterol. However, this information is absent in the summary recommendations, which essentially recite the dogma of *The Establishment*: *reduce dietary fat and eat more carbohydrates.* This pleases the sponsors because the recommendations are often the only parts of such surveys that are read by or taught to busy health professionals. Whereas only the most diligent researchers and medical professionals who read between the survey recommendations will get the whole truth, the vast majority of us will get only the *eat less fat and more carbohydrates* message. The ADA's dietary recommendations have been widely criticized in the diabetic community.[99]

To see why, consider this statement from the American Diabetes Association's 2005 Standards of Medical Care in Diabetes:

> *Low carbohydrate diets are not recommended in the management of diabetes. Although dietary carbohydrate is the major contributor to postprandial glucose concentration, it is an important source of energy, water, soluble vitamins and minerals, and fiber. Thus, [...] a recommended range of carbohydrate intake is 45–65% of*

total calories. [100]

Yes, dietary carbohydrate is a source of energy, but water? Personally I don't find pretzels to be very thirst quenching. The claim that dietary carbohydrate is an important source of soluble vitamins and minerals exemplifies a form of sugarcoating known as manufacturing facts, or simply *Manufacting*. Dietary carbohydrate is *not* an important source of vitamins or minerals. Vitamins and minerals come from nutritious foods, some of which happen to contain carbohydrates (e.g. vegetables) while others don't (e.g. beef). Cookies, crackers, soda, and rice cakes are loaded with carbohydrates but are *not* important sources of vitamins and minerals.

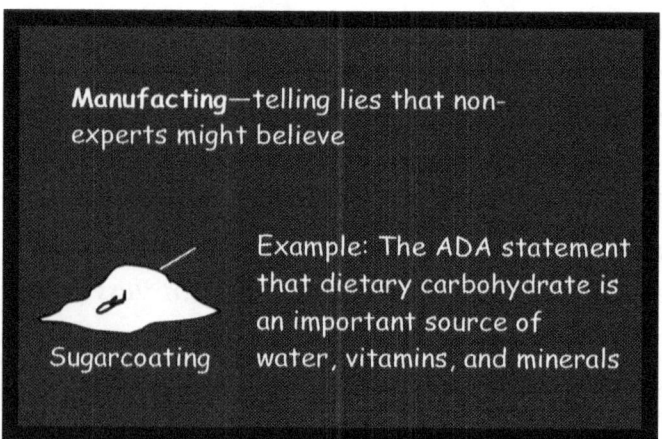

Chalkboard 4.3: Definition of Manufacting

The ADA goes on to say:

In addition, because the brain and central nervous system have an absolute requirement for glucose as an energy source, restricting total carbohydrate to <130 g/day is not recommended. [101]

This is just another example of *Ignorisolation* sugarcoating.

The statement draws your focus to the brain's preference for glucose but leaves out the pertinent fact that *you don't have to eat carbohydrates to make glucose.* Your body can create glucose from protein or fat. This is why your brain doesn't die if you go a day without carbohydrates and why Eskimos can live for months on a diet of fish and seal meat.

List of 2003 ADA Corporate Sponsors

Aventis Pharmaceuticals	Discovery Health Channel
BD Consumer Healthcare	Ebony Magazine
Bristol-Myers Squibb Company	EMD Pharmaceuticals
Eli Lilly and Company	General Mills, Inc.
GlaxoSmithKline	Goldman Sachs and Company
Johnson & Johnson	Health Magazine
Lifescan, Inc., a Johnson & Johnson company	Hershey Foods
Novartis Pharmaceuticals Corporation	Home Diagnostics, Inc.
Novo Nordisk Pharmaceuticals	Liberty Medical Supply
Pfizer Inc	MedWise, Inc.
Takeda Pharmaceuticals North America, Inc.	Merck/Schering-Plough Pharmaceuticals
AstraZeneca	Metrika, Inc.
Medtronic MiniMed	Murray Sugar Free Cookies
Merck & Co., Inc.	Nestle USA, Inc.
Roche Diagnostics Corporation	Ocean Spray Cranberries, Inc.
Abbott Laboratories, Inc., MediSense Products	Olivio Premium Products
Abbott Laboratories, Ross Product Division	Ortho Biotech Products, L.P.
Bayer Corporation	Pacific Cycles, Inc.
Kraft Foods	People Weekly Magazine
McNeil Nutritionals	Performance Bicycles, Inc.
Merisant U.S., Inc.	Roche Pharmaceuticals
Tenet Healthcare Foundation	Safeguard Medical Devices
TheraSense, Inc.	Sankyo Pharmaceuticals, Inc.
Abbott Laboratories	Schering-Plough HealthCare Products, Inc.
Coca Cola Company	Specialty Brands of America
Coolbrands International, Inc.	US Den Tek
CVS/pharmacy	Veryfine Products
Dermik Laboratories, Inc.	Voortman Cookies Limited
	Yahoo!

Table 4.1: List of 2003 ADA corporate sponsors[102]

In 2001, when higher fat, reduced carbohydrate diets like Atkins and The Zone started becoming popular, the nutrition committee of the American Heart Association (AHA) jumped into action issuing a Science Advisory Warning.[103] Regarding the popular high-protein diets the committee stated the following:

1. *Such diets may produce short-term weight loss through dehydration.*

2. *Weight loss may also occur through caloric restriction resulting from the fact that the diets are relatively unpalatable.*

3. *Any improvement in blood cholesterol levels and insulin management would be due to weight loss, not the change in composition.*

4. *A very high-protein diet is especially risky for patients with diabetes because it can speed the progression of diabetic kidney disease.*

5. *The high fat content may be harmful to the cardiovascular system in the long run.*

A closer look at this "warning" reveals that the first three items are not actually warning you about anything; they are saying (1) you won't lose fat, only water (2) if you do lose fat it's because the food tasted so bad that you ate less, and (3) any health improvements are due to fat loss, not because you cut carbs. Making such bold yet unsupported assertions solely to discredit an opposing idea is a method of sugarcoating called *Alarmism*.

The statement about protein in item four employs more *Alarmism*. Whereas high protein intake may present a risk for the one in six type 2 diabetics already suffering from kidney disease, it is not "especially risky" for the other five of six who aren't. "High levels of dietary protein do not cause kidney disease in diabetics or anyone else," remarks endocrinologist and long-time complication-free diabetic Dr. Richard K. Bernstein. Even the American

Diabetes Association, a card-carrying member of *The Establishment*, says, "For persons with diabetes, there is no evidence to suggest that usual protein intake (15–20% of total daily energy) should be modified if renal function is normal."[104] While there is strong consensus that elevated blood sugar is *the* underlying pathology in diabetic kidney disease (that's why it's called *diabetic* kidney disease, not *too-much-protein* kidney disease), the AHA still warns against replacing carbohydrates with protein. Sadly, heeding the AHA's sugarcoated warning about dietary protein could put the majority of type 2 diabetics at greater risk for the very complication it warns about: diabetic kidney disease.

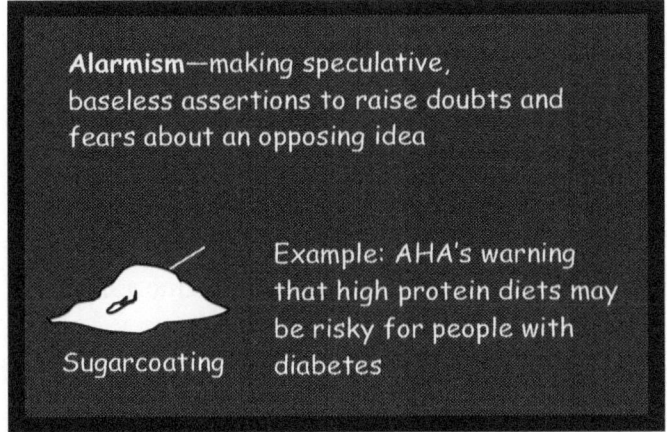

Chalkboard 4.4: Definition of Alarmism

Item 5 speculates that "in the long run" the high fat content of the controlled carbohydrate diet may increase the risk for coronary heart disease (CHD). However, as we've learned, good health is not as simple as limiting a single nutrient or improving a single risk factor. By appealing to the Diet-Heart Hypothesis, item five employs *Ignorisolation*; it focuses on the relationship between dietary fat and LDL cholesterol and ignores all other risk factors for heart disease.

When it comes to risk factors for heart disease, every dietary camp with an ideology to uphold employs it's own form of *Ignorisolation*. Take a look at how each camp explains their diet's effect on CHD risk factors.

- *The Establishment* credits the low fat diet for improving LDL cholesterol, but attributes any improvements on the low carb diet to weight loss, not the reduction in carbs.
- The *Carbophobes* credit the low carb diet for improving blood sugar, blood pressure, triglycerides, and HDL cholesterol. They only talk about LDL cholesterol in the context of the HDL/LDL ratio, which, they claim, improves on the low carb diet.
- The *Low Fat Fundamentalists* trumpet how their diet lowers LDL and say that HDL is not important when you lower your LDL.
- The *Mods* just shake their heads and encourage us to live more like the Greeks, who have a low incidence of heart disease.

The superiority of the Greek (aka Mediterranean) diet was suggested in 1970 by the Seven Countries Study and then demonstrated in the 1990s by the Lyon Diet Heart Study.[105,106] The study involved 605 heart attack survivors, half of whom were instructed to follow a high fat Mediterranean Diet, while the other half were asked to follow the American Heart Association's low fat "prudent" diet. After four years, there were only fourteen cardiac events in the Mediterranean diet group compared to forty-four in the prudent group.[107] Because of this large, statistically significant difference, continuing the trial was considered unethical and the trial was stopped.

The evidence from the Lyon Diet Heart study boldly

contradicts *The Establishment's* low fat message and is so marked that it cannot be refuted. However, it can be sugarcoated with a touch of *Manufacting* to make the AHA diet look like a winner. Although the authors of the Lyon Study publication clearly describe the prudent diet as "close to the step 1 American Heart Association prudent diet," the AHA claims the opposite, saying that the Mediterranean diet used in the study is "consistent with the American Heart Association Eating Plan for Healthy Americans" while the prudent diet is not. [108,109]

Corporate sponsorship appears to be the driving force behind the sugarcoated messages that come from *The Establishment* and mislead the public into making poor health choices. Take for example the American Heart Association's "Heart Check" program, which certifies "heart healthy" foods. Among the benefits to consumers of this program the AHA touts:

1. *It's trustworthy. You can count on the information because it comes from America's most reliable source of heart-health information, the American Heart Association.*

2. *It identifies heart-healthy foods. You know that any product you choose that bears our Food Certification heart-check mark has passed its nutritional guidelines.*

To qualify for AHA certification, a food product must:

- be low in fat, saturated fat, sodium, and cholesterol
- have at least ten percent of the daily value of one or more of vitamin A, vitamin C, calcium, iron or fiber

and the company that markets the product must:

- pay the AHA thousands of dollars
- not be a tobacco company

For a first-year fee and annual renewal fee of thousands of

dollars per product, food companies may have their products certified and receive the privilege to use the AHA's red heart with white check logo on their product's label — as long as the company isn't Kraft foods, which is owned by Philip Morris, Inc., a tobacco company. So, while Cocoa Puffs®, Cookie Crisp®, and Count Chocula® can be certified "heart healthy" products, the Kraft Foods products Post Grape Nuts®, Post Shredded Wheat®, and Post 100% Bran® may not. According to the AHA, exclusion of tobacco companies is another benefit to consumers because it makes the program "socially responsible."

Given the evidence and consensus against refined carbohydrates (even Ornish says they're bad) it doesn't seem socially responsible to certify high sugar and refined carbohydrate foods as heart healthy because they are low in fat and cholesterol (*Ignorisolation*). Doing so is profitable, however. The AHA has used its position as "the nation's most trusted source for information on nutrition and heart health" (their self description) to earn revenue selling a marketing advantage to select corporations. Their heart check label, like most of the advice coming from *The Establishment*, is in line with marketing objectives and out of step with nutritional science.

Programs like the AHA heart check program, the USDA Food Guide Pyramid, and the U.S. government's failure to recommend a daily allowance for sugar reveal *The Establishment's* focus on fat and blind eye toward refined carbohydrates. While all the other dietary camps explicitly warn against the over-consumption of refined carbohydrates, programs of *The Establishment*, like the USDA Food Guide Pyramid, ADA dietary recommendations, and AHA heart check program, give their blessing to low fat junk food, regardless of sugar content. Next, we shall look at the refreshingly un-sugarcoated, science-based advice of the *Mods*.

5

The Mods

Team Name: Mods
Team Captain: Dr. Walter Willett
Biggest Fear: Trans fats, refined carbs
Model Food: Olive Oil

The *Mods* are a unique minority in the politically charged food campground. Their views on nutrition are formulated mostly by up-to-date, scientific evidence and, unlike the other groups, *change* as new evidence unfolds. In this sense, the *Mods* are not sugarcoaters; they are the voice of reason and objectivity in the campground. Consider the way the various camps explain the following:

> *Since the beginning of the low fat movement in the*
> *1970's, average fat intake in the U.S. has decreased from*
> *forty percent of total calories to thirty-four percent and*
> *death rates due to heart disease have decreased by about*
> *one-third.*[110,111,112]

The Establishment sees this as evidence for their point of view and directly credits the reduction in dietary fat for the reduced rate of deaths from heart disease.

The *Carbophobes* say that this is just the result of improved life-saving medical procedures, which are much more common today. They point out that, although the *death rate* from heart disease decreased, the *incidence* of heart disease has not changed.[113]

The *Low Fat Fundamentalists* aren't surprised that the incidence of heart disease hasn't changed; they believe thirty-four percent fat is still far too much fat to have a positive impact.

The *Mods* take a broader look at *all* the data. They cite the relevant facts ignored by all the other groups:

- While the *percentage* of calories from fat has gone down, *total* fat consumption along with total consumption of calories has increased.[114]

- Between 1970 and 1997 the US food supply increased by 500 calories per day per capita.[115]

- During that period consumption of soft drinks rose from 24.3 gallons per capita to 53 gallons.[116] That's two 2-liter bottles per week per man, woman, child and baby.

- By 1997 Americans were consuming 154 pounds of added sugar per year, almost a half pound per day.[117]

Remove the *Ignorisolation* in the other camps' arguments and the real problem becomes obvious; we are consuming more calories without a corresponding increase in activity. Thus, the *Mods'* advice is simple: eat less and exercise more to maintain a healthy weight. For diabetics, weight control is especially important. A review of thirty-three studies showed that even a modest amount of weight loss (less than ten percent) resulted in improved blood sugar control, reduced blood pressure, and reduced cholesterol levels.[118]

Regular exercise is paramount to weight control, and may even be more important than diet. One study comparing the effects of diet and exercise at preventing diabetes found that while those who dieted fared better than those who did nothing, they fared worse than those who just exercised and didn't diet![119] While this may seem remarkable, bear in mind that the diet used in this study was similar to the low-fat prudent diet recommended by the ADA and AHA.

The *Mods'* emphasis on weight control makes a subtle, but most important point—*watch your portions and calories.* This important point is overshadowed in the other camps by sexy "eat all you want, just avoid the evil nutrient" fad diets, sponsor-approved dietary recommendations, and the miniature portion sizes of the Food Guide Pyramid, all of which encourage greater food consumption, not less.

Harvard Medical School's Healthy Eating Pyramid, which was developed by *Mods* team captain Dr. Walter Willett and colleagues, places "Daily Exercise and Weight Control" at its base to indicate the primary importance of caloric balance. Willet and others at the Harvard Medical School developed the Healthy Eating Pyramid to provide a purely science-based alternative to the USDA Food Guide Pyramid (1992 version).

Willett, like many nutritionists, felt that the Food Guide Pyramid was severely flawed. To prove this, Willett and colleagues performed a study to test whether people who follow the recommendations of the USDA Pyramid are healthier than those who don't. Using the USDA's own Healthy Eating Index, a measure of how well a diet conforms to the Food Guide Pyramid, the researchers showed that, among more than 100,000 subjects over a period of eight to twelve years, those with the highest Healthy Eating Index scores were no better off than those with the lowest scores.[120,121]

Despite this result and over a decade of evidence, the government did not change its guidelines until 2005. However, the new 2005 Food Guide Pyramid still maintains its classic pro-dairy, pro-grain, anti-fat, and soft-on-sugar message. According to Willett, "They say, 'You really need a high level of proof to change the recommendations,' which is ironic, because they never had a high level of proof to set them."[122]

The *Mods* know that outdated messages from *The Establishment* such as "all fats are bad" and "all complex carbohydrates are good" have withered in light of current evidence. They are astutely aware of the numerous failed attempts to show a correlation between a high fat diets and negative health outcomes. They know the evidence shows no correlation between dietary fat and heart disease or obesity. [123,124,125] Dr. Willet reports, "Diets high in fat do not appear to be the primary cause of the high prevalence of excess body fat in our society, and reductions in fat will not be a solution."[126] Moreover, Willett states, "The emphasis on total fat reduction has been a serious distraction in efforts to control obesity and improve health in general."[127]

However, while the *Mods* challenge outdated theories on fat, they are not trying to start a revolution and don't entertain any notions that eliminating one nutrient from the diet is the key to good health. Rather, their advice distinguishes between different types of fats and carbohydrates, encouraging greater consumption of the healthy types and reduction of the more harmful types.

What are the healthy types? Well, let's start with fat. Fats are nutrients necessary to ensure proper growth, brain development, construction of cell membranes and hormones, and other essential bodily functions. When we say "different types of fats," we are really talking about different types of fatty acids, the molecules that join in threes to make fat molecules, also known as triglycerides.

You can visualize a fatty acid as a string of pearls, anywhere from three to thirty pearls long, with each pearl having exactly two spots for a decoration to be attached. If every pearl in the string has both decorations attached (chemically, every carbon atom has bonded to two hydrogen atoms), then our fatty acid is said to be *saturated*. If all but one pearl is fully decorated, then we have a *monounsaturated* fatty acid. If multiple pearls are missing decorations, then we have a *polyunsaturated* fatty acid. Put any three strings of pearls together and you have a triglyceride (a fat molecule consisting of three fatty acids attached to a glycerol molecule) as illustrated in Chalkboard 5.1.

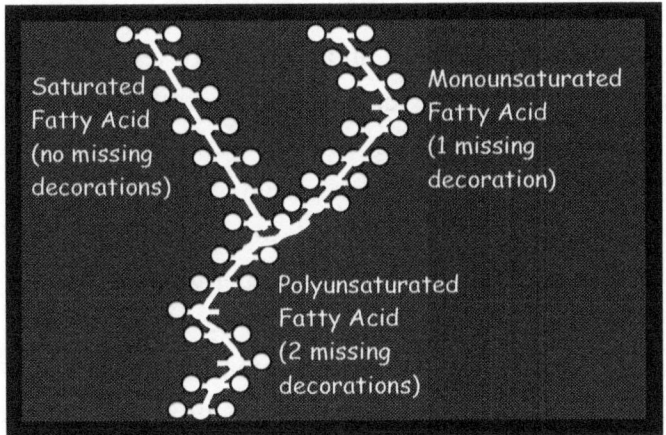

Chalkboard 5.1: A Triglyceride consisting of one of each type of fatty acid.

These three general classifications are the ones most commonly used to identify fat types, however within each there exist many different types of fatty acids. Biochemists have identified and studied every type of fatty acid they can find to understand the function of each one. Thanks to their work we know, for example, that the fatty acid Docosahexaenoic acid

(DHA) is used in the formation of membranes in the brain and eye, and of another fatty acid, Eicosapentaenoic acid (EPA), which is used to make hormones.

DHA and EPA both belong to a family of fats that is currently receiving a lot of attention from nutritionists: the omega-3 fatty acids. The term omega-3 was undoubtedly coined by a scientist (scientists are infatuated with the Greek alphabet) to indicate where the first "kink" in a fatty acid molecule occurs. As shown in Chalkboard 5.1, kinks occur at places where pearls are missing decorations (i.e., where carbons are missing hydrogens). When the first pearl missing a decoration is third from the end, we call it an omega-3; if it is sixth, it is an omega-6 and so on.

Omega-3 fatty acids are of interest because they have been shown to improve triglyceride and cholesterol levels and may have a significant role in the prevention of coronary heart disease.[128,129] In fact, clinical trials have demonstrated that eating omega-3 fats is as good or better at preventing heart attacks than ingesting lipid-lowering drugs.[130,131,132,133] Omega-3 fatty acids are known to help reduce inflammation and it is believed that a deficiency of omega-3s in the western diet is playing a role in the rising rate of inflammatory disorders. Thus, many nutritionists are recommending supplements, such as fish oil and flaxseed oil, which are high in omega-3s.

The Lyon Diet Heart Study showed that the Mediterranean diet, which is high in omega-3 and monounsaturated fatty acids, is superior to the low fat American Heart Association prudent diet in preventing heart disease.[134] Thus the *Mods* recommend we eat more like Mediterraneans, by replacing carbohydrates with good types of fats. Numerous studies have shown that doing so improves blood lipid profiles, reduces fasting glucose levels, enables better weight loss maintenance, and reduces the risk of heart disease and diabetes.[135,136,137,138,139,140] The *Mods* discourage low fat and no fat versions of normal foods in which heart healthy unsaturated fats are removed and replaced with carbohydrates (typically sugar). For example, they shun fat-free salad dressings because they know that carotenes and other important nutrients in the salad require fat for transport and storage. Olive oil, made up of 70% monounsaturated fat, is the salad dressing of choice in the Mediterranean diet and accordingly has become the *Nectar of the Mods.*

Other good sources of unsaturated fats include nuts, seeds, avocados, vegetable oils, and fatty fish. Even a juicy steak can be a source of "heart-healthy" (i.e. lipid-lowering) fats. As science writer Gary Taubes points out, fifty-five percent of the fat in beef is healthy unsaturated fat and fifteen percent is the saturated fat stearic acid, which has a neutral effect on blood lipids.[141]

Whereas health information has been dominated by the ambitious speculation that saturated fat is unhealthy because it raises total cholesterol, very little has been said about another type of dietary fat, trans fatty acids. However, that is starting to change. Researchers at the Harvard School of Public Health have performed studies in which thousands of participants were surveyed about their diets and tracked for health outcomes over several years. Whereas the investigators found a weak positive correlation between dietary saturated fat and heart disease they found a strong relationship between the intake of trans fatty acids and heart disease. Just a two percent increment in trans fatty acids was associated with a ninety-three percent increase in relative risk![142,143]

Trans fatty acids, also known as trans fats, are fats that are, most commonly, formed in the process of partially hydrogenating vegetable oils to make them solid at room temperature. Partial hydrogenation can change the structure of the fatty acid into what is called a *trans* configuration (picture a tangled string of pearls). Instead of eliminating trans fats as waste, the body uses them in place of normal fats to build cell membranes. This can affect the vital process of transporting nutrients and waste across the cell membrane. Trans fats also block utilization of essential fatty acids and are associated with a number of severe health problems including heart disease, cancer, and diabetes.[144,145,146,147] Some adverse effects related to trans fatty acids are listed in Chalkboard 5.2.[148]

Effects of Trans Fatty Acid Consumption

* Worsens cholesterol profile
* Lowers immune response
* Increases levels of abnormal sperm
* Inhibits conversion of essential fatty acids
* Alters membrane transport and fluidity
* Potentiates free radical formation
* Precipitates asthma
* Decreases visual acuity in infants
* Low birth weight

Chalkboard 5.2: Effects of Trans Fatty Acid Consumption

For these reasons the *Mods* recommend eliminating or reducing as much as possible the intake of trans fats. For over twenty years researchers like Dr. Mary Enig have been warning of the dangers of trans fats and finally *The Establishment* is acknowledging the evidence. The Federal Dietary Guidelines for Americans recommend reducing the intake of trans fat and the FDA now requires that information on trans fatty acids be provided on the Nutrition Facts panel of food labels. While the labeling requirement will help consumers to determine what's in their margarine or favorite snack food, it won't help with fast foods and over-the-counter doughnuts, which generally do not come with nutrition facts labels.

Heat and oxygen also damage fats, making them unhealthy for consumption. Dr. Schwarzbein recommends using only oils that have been expeller pressed or cold pressed (e.g. extra virgin olive oil) and only cooking with oils high in saturated or monounsaturated fats (e.g. butter or olive oil) because these are more stable at higher temperatures than polyunsaturates. You will find polyunsaturated fats that have been "refined" to withstand heat, but this process causes them to lose most of their healthy omega-3 fatty acids according to lipids expert Mary Enig.

Thus, it appears that the best way to get fats is to consume them in their natural or near-natural forms. Using olive oil and/or flaxseeds to dress a salad, snacking on raw nuts and avocados, and enjoying fresh cold-water fish are ways to get the right kinds of fats in your diet. According to the *Mods*, health has little to do with how much fat one eats but very much to do with the type of fat.

The *Mods* offer similar advice for carbohydrates. Carbohydrates in the diet ultimately provide us with glucose, the currency of energy in the body. Glucose and its sibling molecules, called monosaccharides, are the building blocks of carbohydrates such as sugar and starch. Whereas table sugar is made up of only two monosaccharides, starches may contain thousands. Some starches have a bushy structure with several side branches (these are called *amylopectins*) while others have a straight and long structure (these are called *amyloses*), These two forms are important because the structure of a starch gives us a good idea of the impact it will have on blood sugar.

As important as a carbohydrate's structure is the package that it comes in. Most carbohydrates found in nature come packaged with a generous helping of fiber and nutrients. For example, a grain of whole wheat in its natural form contains a nutrient-rich core called the *germ*, surrounded by a starchy layer called the *endosperm*, which is encased in a fibrous shell called the *bran*. The process of refining flour involves extracting just the endosperm, leaving the germ and bran, along with a bunch of vitamins, minerals, fiber, unsaturated fats, and other phytochemicals behind. The resulting product is typically so nutritionally deficient that federal law requires it to be enriched or fortified with vitamins and minerals. Fortifying a product amounts to spraying a liquid multivitamin supplement on it. To your body, eating a slice of bread made from enriched whole-wheat flour is not unlike eating a chocolate chip cookie with a low-grade vitamin pill. You might as well enjoy the cookie and take a better vitamin.

Similarly, refined products made from fruits and vegetables often suffer nutritional losses. When raw fruit is processed into fruit juices and fruit cocktails, a substantial loss of fiber and vitamins occurs. To make matters worse, sugar or high-fructose corn syrup is often added. High fructose corn syrup and sugar are themselves examples of vegetables refined to a nutritionless state.

Refined carbohydrates not only lack nutrients, but because they lack the fiber that comes with carbohydrates in their natural forms they are converted to blood glucose and triglycerides more rapidly and make you hungry again sooner. Fiber, which is indigestible by humans, appears to slow down the process of carbohydrate absorption. Increased intake of dietary fiber is associated with a reduction of triglycerides and improved glycemic control in diabetics.[149,150] Moreover, researchers have found some association between high fiber diets and reduced risk of diabetes and heart disease.[151,152,153]

The *Mods* are interested in the connection between health

outcomes and the consumption of foods that raise blood sugar quickly. Rather than pay homage to an outdated theory about "complex" carbohydrates, they have experimentally measured how different foods affect blood sugar. The glycemic index (GI) is the metric they use; the higher the GI number, the greater the impact the food has on blood glucose. The GI for a specific food is determined by feeding several subjects a portion of the food containing fifty grams of digestible carbohydrate (not counting fiber) and measuring their glucose levels over the next two hours. On another day, the same subjects consume fifty grams of pure glucose and the same measurements are taken. The GI value for the food is computed by comparing the two sets of results with pure glucose being assigned a reference GI of 100. Chalkboard 5.3 gives the experimentally determined glycemic index of a few foods.[154]

Glycemic Index of Selected Foods	
Food	GI
Kellogg's Corn Flakes	92
Rice cake (low-amylose)	87
White Bread	70
Rice cake (high-amylose)	61
Kellogg's Frosties	55
75% Whole-grain Bread	48
Whole Milk	27
Kidney Beans	23
Peanuts	14

Chalkboard 5.3: Glycemic Index of Selected Foods

From this small sampling of the foods we can make several observations that are generally true with few or no exceptions. First, we see the top spots on the list being held by many of the so-called "complex" carbohydrates recommended by *The*

Establishment. In addition to rice cakes and Corn Flakes, you will find potatoes, breads, muffins, cereals, and other staples of the Food Guide Pyramid having high GI values. Down at the bottom of the list we find beans and nuts. Legumes such as beans and peanuts tend to be higher in amyloses and lower in amylopectins than other "complex" carbohydrates. It is believed that they turn into blood sugar more slowly because amyloses (the long straight structures) take longer to digest than amylopectins (the bushy structures). While this theory may seem reminiscent of the old "complex vs. simple" hypothesis, it has one striking difference: it is supported by scientific evidence. In feeding experiments, high-amylose versions of a food consistently have lower glycemic index values than their low-amylose counterparts.[155]

Second, we see that while white bread has a high glycemic index, whole-grain bread falls in the low GI range. This may be due to the added fiber because fibrous foods tend to have lower GI scores.[156] The GI of pure glucose taken with fiber is about forty percent lower than without (i.e., 60 versus 100). Though there have been mixed results in some GI studies comparing fiber-enriched breads to their "fiber-challenged" counterparts, the sum of GI data suggests that fiber, especially that from carbohydrates in their natural form, slows down the rise in blood glucose.

Next, we observe that whole milk comes in toward the bottom of the GI scale. Unlike starches, the carbohydrate in milk comes in the form of lactose, a very small carbohydrate molecule that most people over age two have trouble digesting. Half of lactose is a sugar called galactose, which has to be converted to glucose and is digested more slowly. This may explain why whole milk has a lower GI than Soy milk (27 versus 44), which contains no lactose. However, the GI of pure lactose is also considerably higher than whole milk, so the low GI of milk can't be completely attributed to lactose. Whole milk contains a fair portion of fat and protein, which can slow digestion and increase insulin response. Studies suggest that having fat or protein with a carbohydrate lowers the GI.[157] Whole milk has a GI about twenty percent lower than skim milk and the GI of buttered white bread is about sixteen percent lower than plain white bread.

Finally, we observe that *Kellogg's Frosties* (the European/Australian brand name for those g-r-r-r-eat sugarcoated corn flakes) have a lower GI than plain old unsweetened *Kellogg's Corn Flakes*. While it is not yet clear why this is, the data does suggest that sugar is no worse than refined flour in elevating blood glucose levels. In fact, pure table sugar has a GI lower than white bread, as do *Coca-Cola* and honey. This may be because these sweets all contain high amounts of fructose, which must be converted to glucose. The GI of pure fructose is 19, roughly eighty percent lower than pure glucose.

By using the same amount of carbohydrate for each food tested, the GI provides an excellent reference for comparison. However, the index does not take into account the most important factor in elevating blood sugar: the *amount* of carbohydrates eaten. Based on GI alone, one might conclude that a slice of chocolate cake with frosting (with its GI of 38) is a better dessert choice than a slice of watermelon (with a GI of 72). Such thinking doesn't take into account that a single serving slice of the cake contains roughly *ten times* more carbohydrates than a single serving of watermelon. Thus, serving for serving, watermelon doesn't raise blood sugar nearly as much as cake. Similarly, while cooked carrots and baked potatoes have roughly the same GI, a serving of potato contains far more carbs than a normal serving of carrots and thus has a much greater effect on blood sugar.

Because factoring in grams of carbs and GI can be tedious and error-prone, the *glycemic load* scale was developed. The glycemic load is just the number of carbohydrates in a serving multiplied by the glycemic index and divided by one hundred. It is similar to a carb count in that you can add glycemic loads together to determine the overall load for a meal or a day. The glycemic load of our selected foods is shown in Chalkboard 5.4 below.[158]

With the carb count factored in, the list, now reordered by glycemic load value, shifts around a bit. We find carb-dense *Frosties* working their way toward the top and whole milk, which has some fat and protein, dropping further toward the bottom. In general, a food having a significant fraction of calories from fat and protein will have fewer carbs in a serving and thus a lower glycemic load than a pure-carb food. This is a good rule of thumb to use when putting together meals, especially when you don't have a glycemic load table handy.

Glycemic Load of Selected Foods	
Food	GL
Kellogg's Corn Flakes	23.2
Rice cake (low-amylose)	16.1
Kellogg's Frosties	14.4
Rice cake (high-amylose)	11.3
White Bread	9.4
75% Whole-grain Bread	6.1
Kidney Beans	5.5
Whole Milk	3.8
Peanuts	0.6

Chalkboard 5.4: Glycemic Load of Selected Foods

Maintaining a good balance of carbohydrates, fat, and protein in every meal is the fundamental principle of Dr. Barry Sears' popular Zone weight loss diet. Although the Zone and South Beach diets have been labeled "low carb" diets, they don't belong in the

Carbophobes camp. They are balanced diets based on current nutritional evidence without sugarcoating, which puts them squarely in the Mods camp.

Despite all its utility, the low glycemic index diet is not recommended by the American Diabetes Association. Why? Because, they say, it is too complicated for the health professional, let alone the diabetic patient. This is just more *Alarmism* sugarcoating. The claim is purely speculative and there is evidence to refute it. When compared to the carbohydrate exchange diet advocated by the ADA, the glycemic index was no more difficult to implement and produced better results for children with type 1 diabetes. The children who were given low-GI dietary advice had significantly lower HbA1c scores and fewer hyperglycemic episodes than their counterparts on the ADA diet.[159] However, just because kids can understand it, one shouldn't assume that adults and health professionals can.

The glycemic load is a handy tool for estimating how much a meal is going to raise blood sugar. If you are eating different kinds of foods, you can, in theory, just add their glycemic loads together. However, accuracy is limited because the glycemic load can change depending on how the food is prepared, how quickly it is eaten, how much it is chewed before swallowing, and the levels of vitamins and minerals in your body. The published glycemic load numbers themselves have some margin for error because every subject tested is different. Diabetics are especially unique when it comes to blood sugar response to food. As always, recognize that your meter is the ultimate authority on how food affects *your* blood sugar and let it be your guide.

After your meter, the best source of unbiased information is the *Mods*. Their message is consistent and evidence-based: get more exercise, fiber, and omega-3 fatty acids and cut out refined carbohydrates and trans fatty acids. For all their political positioning, none of the other camps fundamentally disagrees with any of these recommendations. They just choose to focus elsewhere. Fortunately, the *Mods* don't. When it comes to diet, the *Mods* are your ticket to get past the sugarcoating.

In a sea of sugarcoated books on diet there are a few good ones written by members of the *Mods* camp. Dr. Walter Willett's *Eat, Drink, and Be Healthy: The Harvard Medical School Guide to Healthy Eating*, is an example of a science-based, sugar-free view of nutrition. *The Schwarzbein Principle: The Truth About Losing Weight, Being Healthy, and Feeling Younger* by Dr. Diana Schwarzbein and Nancy Deville provides some eye-opening and effective advice on diet. Perhaps the most scientific, myth-debunking book on dietary fat is *Know Your Fats: The Complete Primer for Understanding the Nutrition of Fats, Oils and Cholesterol*, by Mary Enig, Ph.D. These books are all written by knowledgeable scientists and rated excellent by reviewers on Amazon.com. Dr. Barry Sears' series of books about *The Zone* diet, while grounded in good science, are not as highly acclaimed by reviewers, however. One thing different about *The Zone* series is that companies such as ZonePerfect and Zone Labs Inc. have capitalized on the popularity of the diet to sell a complete line of "Zone-compliant" shakes, bars, and nutritional supplements. Selling dietary substitutes and supplements is a multi-billion dollar business and accordingly is ripe with sugarcoating. The next section of this book examines this sugarcoating and provides a science-based look at dietary substitutes and supplements.

Part II: Supplements and Substitutes

Part one of this book revealed how the sugarcoating of dietary information is responsible for the inconsistency and controversy surrounding the most fundamental questions about diet. It showed how to distinguish corporate marketing from science-based advice and delivered science-based answers to the controversial questions. You've probably known these answers all along, but the sugarcoating made you forget them. You didn't need a food pyramid or a fad diet book to tell you it was better to have a grilled chicken salad than a slice of sugar-free chocolate cake; you just needed to have a few myths debunked.

In that vein, we now turn our attention towards the world of substitute foods and dietary supplements. Diet shakes, nutrition bars, vitamin drinks and good old-fashioned vitamin pills are enormous sellers in the United States, where putting synthetic products into our bodies is the rule and consuming natural ones the exception. We consume synthetic foods, synthetic drinks, synthetic vitamins, and synthetic drugs with such frequency that we view anything that isn't artificial as special and deserving of labels such as "all natural" or "contains no artificial ingredients." We label foods that haven't been genetically modified, shot with hormones, or sprayed with chemicals as "organic" and even have a "real" seal for dairy products to indicate when they're not synthetic. Even cigarette manufacturers make it a point to let you know that their brand is made from "all natural" tobacco.

If all natural is a selling point, does this mean that synthetic is bad? Of course not. We have government agencies looking out for us to ensure that every synthetic product we put in our bodies is safe ... well, perhaps not. The following chapters uncover the reality about food substitutes and dietary supplements and reveal the types of sugarcoating used to promote the consumption of these products.

6

Food Substitutes

If you flip through the pages of any diabetes magazine you won't find many ads espousing the wonders of broccoli, spinach, or peanuts. The foods advertised to us are always diet soft drinks, nutrition bars, shakes, and sugar-free and fat-free desserts. Free samples of these are routinely given out at health fairs, diabetes events, and support groups. Your certified diabetes educator has an endless supply of these. Your well-meaning friends and relatives often bring them to social engagements so you don't feel left out. Fast food, junk food, snack food, and soda are so ingrained in American culture that giving all of them up, even when faced with diabetes, can seem like an impossible task. Even when the long-term consequences are known, short-term pleasure and/or convenience make poor eating choices all too easy to make.

Enter the benevolent food manufacturers, who bring fantastic news: Americans need not worry because their substitute junk foods are healthy! Now more than ever, health conscious Americans are happily getting their nutrition from meal replacement bars and shakes, fully believing that these products are healthy and fit their busy lifestyle. Although these products often amount to little more than synthetic food with added multivitamins we want to believe that they are good for us. Doing so is very liberating. With attractive marketing slogans like "pleasure without guilt" and "have your cake and eat it too" the food industry is squarely targeting our vulnerability to junk food, assuring us that they have lifted our burden of making disciplined choices simply by exorcising the "evil nutrient" from our junk food.

Within this hopeful message, however, lies an obvious contradiction. The food industry recognizes not one but two villains—fat and carbohydrates—yet never at the same time. Whether fats or carbs are the real enemy is up to the customer and depends on which line of sugarcoating she believes. The food industry doesn't care because it plays both sides. Whether it be low carb, low fat, fat-free, or sugar-free, there is a guilt-free ice cream for everyone.

To make a substitute taste better, manufacturers often play the "compensation game," removing one evil nutrient while adding more of the other. Low carb products often contain more fat than their regular counterparts while reduced fat products almost always contain more carbohydrates (see Figure 6.1).

If fat is truly the evil nutrient, then low carb substitutes should be worse for you than regular junk food. Similarly, if carbs are the real enemy, then low fat substitutes should be less healthy. Which is it? The grocery store is filled with many examples of this contradiction; low carb and low fat substitutes, each containing more of the other's villain, are often positioned right next to each other on the shelf. Even when a substitute doesn't contain more of the other's presumed evil nutrient, the impression that it is a "free" food can lead to over-consumption.

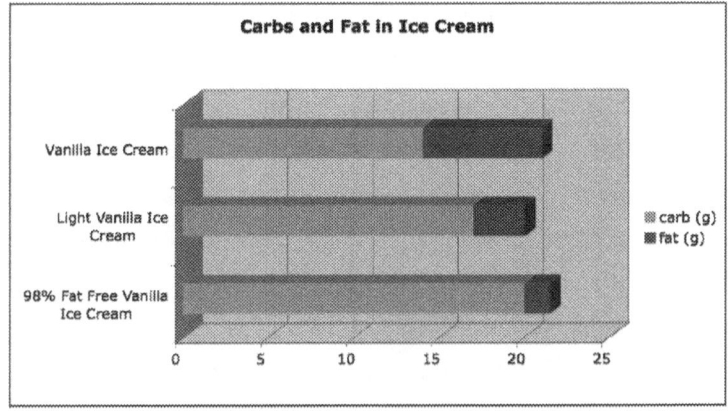

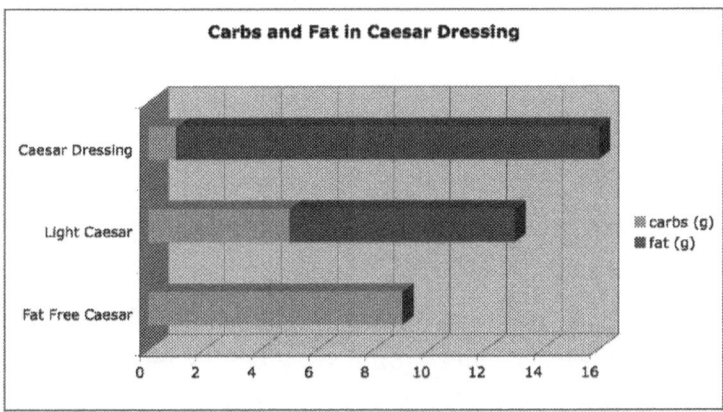

Figure 6.1: The compensation game: less fat equals more carbohydrates

The promise of low fat substitutes is that they are a good way to curb fat intake and thus make you lighter and healthier. Member organizations of *The Establishment* publish statements like, "Moderate use of low-calorie, reduced-fat foods, combined with low total energy intake, could potentially promote dietary intake consistent with the objectives of Healthy People 2010 and the 2005 Dietary Guidelines for Americans."[160] Amidst all the non-commitant words like "moderate," "could," and "potentially," the phrase contains a key stipulation, *"combined with a low energy intake*," that pinpoints a major reason why reduced fat substitutes are ineffective at weight control and have no proven health benefit: our bodies play the compensation game too. Studies show that whereas low fat and fat-free substitutes can decrease dietary fat intake, this comes with a corresponding increase in calories from protein and carbohydrates.[161,162] Since the introduction of low fat foods Americans have decreased the percentage of calories from dietary fat not by consuming less fat, but by consuming more calories overall.[163,164] This is not surprising since extra carbohydrate calories are often right there in the reduced fat substitute.

The claim that low fat junk foods are healthy is another example of *Guiltabsolution* sugarcoating. Studies have repeatedly shown that replacing carbohydrates in the diet with unsaturated fatty acids improves blood lipids and reduces risk for heart disease, stroke, and diabetes.[165,166,167,168,169] Nevertheless, makers of low fat substitutes do the opposite; they remove healthy unsaturated fats from their products and replace them with carbohydrates. Remember the oversimplified mantra, "eat less fat and you will lower your risk for heart disease"? The lack of distinction among the different types of fat was necessary for the success of low fat substitutes because if consumers could make this distinction there would be almost nothing to cut out and no product to market. Most foods contain relatively little saturated fat, so it is common in creating low fat substitutes to remove far more unsaturated fats than saturated fats. In low fat peanut butter, for example, four grams of healthy unsaturated fat are removed for every gram of saturated fat purged. In low fat mayonnaise the ratio is almost seven to one. Ironically, the indiscriminate removal of healthy unsaturated fats and their replacement with carbohydrates makes low fat substitutes worse for your cholesterol than the full fat, lower carbohydrate versions.[170] This is the danger in *Guiltabsolution* sugarcoating.

Recently, concern about both fat and carbohydrate content has led to the development of substitute foods that are low in both. However, removing both fat and carbohydrate from a junk food leaves nothing to give it taste and the whole purpose of junk food is to taste good. To remedy this problem the food industry has developed nutrient substitutes, such as artificial sweeteners, sugar alcohols, and artificial fat, which add flavor to food substitutes that have been depleted of sugar and fat. These chemical cousins to the real thing often contain few or no calories because your body doesn't digest them very well. Although your digestive enzymes may not recognize them, your tongue does, and that is the secret to making delicious, "guilt-free" substitute products. (As we shall see, guilt is still warranted.)

Artificial sweeteners, also called non-nutritive sweeteners because they contain no calories, are often used to sweeten sugar-free products such as diet soda, Jell-o, and cookies. The top artificial sweetener for many years was Aspartame. Aspartame is used in diet soft drinks and hundreds of other products; however, it is not used for baking. Under heat, aspartame breaks down into methanol, which, in the absence of ethanol, further breaks down into the toxic chemicals formaldehyde and formic acid. The manufacturer claims this is not a safety issue because methanol is found in greater quantities in natural foods in our diet. However, natural foods, unlike aspartame, contain enough ethanol to inhibit the breakdown of methanol into toxic chemicals. The FDA has received thousands of documented complaints linking aspartame to ninety-two different disorders including headaches, dizziness, mood disorders, nausea, abdominal pain, change in vision, diarrhea, seizures, and memory loss.[171] There are Internet sites filled with information about the dangers of aspartame and support groups for people who suffer from "aspartame disease." Groups such as the FDA, AMA, and ADA all say aspartame is completely safe and hundreds of studies support their view. However, a disturbing number don't. An unpublished review of aspartame studies concluded that of 166 studies examined, one hundred percent of the industry-funded research affirmed aspartame's safety, whereas ninety-two percent of the independently funded research did not.[172] Whether or not aspartame is safe is really a personal question: *does aspartame cause any problems for me?* If you can tolerate aspartame, go ahead and enjoy a refreshing Diet Coke® ... just make sure you keep it refrigerated. The aspartame in diet cola left at room temperature for seventy days decomposes into more than four times as much formaldehyde than that in refrigerated soda.[173]

Splenda® (a.k.a. sucralose) has recently replaced aspartame as the dominant artificial sweetener. Unlike aspartame, Splenda® is heat stable, so it can be used for baking and is safe in warm soda. Both Coca-Cola® and Pepsi® now offer diet soft drinks sweetened with Splenda®. The marketing slogan for Splenda®, *"Made from sugar, so it tastes like sugar"* has been criticized for creating the false perception that Splenda® is a natural sweetener made from real sugar. Competitors have petitioned the Federal Trade Commission and filed lawsuits claiming that the slogan misleads consumers. Yes, the maker of Splenda® is being sued for *Guiltabsolution* sugarcoating. The ironic thing about this slogan is that the consumer is expected to take comfort in the fact that Splenda® is made from real sugar, the evil nutrient. Splenda® is made from sugar that is chemically modified by replacing hydrogen-oxygen groups with chlorine atoms. It is no more natural than any of the other synthetics approved as artificial sweeteners.

If a natural sugar substitute is what consumers want, then it may seem odd that not one of the FDA approved artificial sweeteners is a natural product. (Possibly related fact: it is very difficult to patent natural products already in the food supply.) Stevia, a natural, zero calorie, extract of the *stevia rebaudiana* shrub, has been used as a natural sweetener for centuries. Because stevia is not approved by the FDA, it can only be sold as a dietary supplement and cannot be labeled as a sweetener. The FDA's curiously aggressive stance toward the importing, marketing, and sales of the natural sweetener, which included confiscating and burning stevia recipe books is well documented.[174,175]

In addition to non-nutritive sweeteners, there is another important class of sweeteners called sugar alcohols. These calorie-containing sweeteners are often found in low "net carb" bars as well as "sugar-free" chocolates, syrups, and hard candies. Products made with sugar alcohols can be labeled "sugar-free" thus giving the impression that they are a "free" food that can be consumed without restraint. This is just *Guiltabsolution* sugarcoating; sugar alcohols contain carbohydrates and calories. Most sugar alcohols are poorly absorbed so they don't raise blood sugar as much or as rapidly as equivalent amounts of glucose or sucrose (table sugar).[176,177,178,179] However, their effect varies greatly depending on the type of sugar alcohol, as shown in Table 6.1. Sugar alcohols typically have about half to three-quarters the calories of sugar, but they also have around half to three-quarters of the sweetness, so it takes roughly the same amount of calories to achieve the same level of sweetness.

Name	Glycemic Index (sugar=65)	Calories/gram (sugar=4)
Erythritol	0	0.2
Isomalt	9	2.1
Lactitol	6	2.0
Maltitol	36	2.7
Mannitol	0	1.5
Polyglycitol	39	2.8
Sorbitol	9	2.5
Xylitol	13	3.0

Table 6.1 Properties of some sugar alcohols. Source: Livesey 2003[180]

Because sugar alcohol substitutes contain significant amounts of carbohydrates and calories, they count, despite what Atkins marketing slogans claim about "net impact" carbs. Not only do these substitutes have a net impact on blood sugar, they have a net impact on your colon; sugar alcohols can give you the runs.[181,182,183] Although product labels carry a warning about the laxative effects of over-consumption, the FDA has not established an acceptable daily intake of sugar alcohols. As with all carbohydrates, let your glucometer guide you in using sugar alcohols.

Now let us turn our attention to the other evil nutrient: fat. Fat is the essence of many foods. It provides the smoothness in cheese, the creaminess in ice cream, the flakiness in piecrust, the softness in cake, the crispness of a cookie, and the golden goodness in fried chicken. Because it is evil, however, the food industry has devoted considerable resources to developing low fat and fat-free substitutes for just about every fat-containing food. This has not been easy. One of the obstacles to acceptance of reduced fat foods is that they are watery and often lacking the flavor and texture provided by natural fat.

Fat substitutes are used to put the goodness of fat back into low fat foods. Often a mixture of different fat substitutes is needed to mimic all facets of the real thing. Each of the different types of fat substitutes has its relative strengths in creating a fat-like taste, aroma, mouth feel, etc. The protein-based and carbohydrate-based substitutes are most often used to imitate the creamy mouth feel of fat. They are used in a variety of foods, including yogurt, ice cream, and milkshakes, sauces, dips, soups, spreads, frostings, frozen desserts, salad dressings, processed meats, baked goods, and sweets. They provide from zero to four calories per gram, depending on their water content and, because they do not contain any oils, they do not work for frying. The fat-based substitutes consist of modified fatty acids that often provide fewer calories than regular fat. They can replace fats and oils in all typical applications, including formulated products, baking and frying.

Partially hydrogenated vegetable oils are commonly used to give a creamy texture and longer shelf life to baked goods. They are used to make artificial butter, also known as margarine, appear more butter-like. Margarine has for many years been marketed as a healthier alternative to butter because it contains less saturated fat. However, the hydrogenated vegetable oils in margarine contain trans fats, which (unlike other fats) are strongly associated with several major health problems including heart disease, cancer, and diabetes.[184,185,186,187]

Olestra is a combination fat substitute made from sugar and fatty acids. The resulting molecule is too large to be absorbed by the digestive tract and thus Olestra provides no calories. Although the FDA has approved Olestra for use in fried snack foods and crackers, it requires supplementation with vitamins A, D, E, and K because Olestra inhibits the absorption of these fat-soluble vitamins. Known side affects of Olestra include anal oil leakage, intestinal discomfort, cramps, and diarrhea. Olestra significantly reduces blood levels of carotenoids, the pigments found in vegetables that protect against chronic diseases.[188,189]

The marketing of junk food made fat-free using Olestra is another case of *Guiltabsolution* sugarcoating. *Mods* captain Dr. Walter Willett predicts that moderate consumption of Olestra would result in thousands of cases of prostate cancer, coronary heart disease, lung cancer, and macular degeneration leading to blindness.[190] He and other prominent nutritionists have called for the revocation of FDA's approval of Olestra. Willett raises the important question, "Isn't it strange to encourage people to gorge on junk food rather than just not eat it?"[191]

Willet's question addresses the main point of this section: junk food is still junk food no matter what chemical gyrations are performed on it or sugarcoated marketing slogans are applied. As we have seen, the notion that substitute junk food is healthy and safe for diabetics is not only false, but dangerous. Modern technology has not absolved us from using self-discipline in making personal choices; it has just given us more options.

Our next chapter deals with synthetic nutrition and the sugarcoating coming from the dietary supplement industry.

7

Dietary Supplements

Nearly a third of the U.S. population uses dietary supplements. While Americans may have the world's most expensive pee, whether or not the supplements make them any healthier is a hotly debated question. Detractors argue that Americans are recklessly over-consuming supplements, which are not proven safe or effective. Proponents counter that supplements are necessary to compensate for our nutrient-deficient diets and a medical system that ignores prevention. Both sides agree that natural foods are the best way to get all the nutrients your body needs, but that's where the agreement ends.

The reality, according to supplement proponents, is that the typical American diet is horribly deficient in vitamins and minerals. Our foods are grown on depleted soils that lack essential nutrients and cooking them further destroys nutrients. Pollution, stress, and aging all increase our nutrition requirements making it even more difficult to meet our needs from a balanced diet alone. A supplement can provide insurance to those who don't always have the time to eat well.

Indeed, supplements, meal replacement bars, and shakes are frequently marketed to those who are "on the go" or have otherwise busy lifestyles. This familiar form of sugarcoating, *Guiltabsolution*, is essentially saying, "It's OK if you're too busy to eat healthy because we've got a pill that will fix everything."

Recommending a pill that is not proven safe or effective goes against the medical precept "first do no harm," argue the detractors. Vitamins are essential but more does not equal better. Excessive doses of a single nutrient can interfere with the functions of other nutrients and may be toxic. The National Academy of Sciences has established a Recommended Dietary Allowance (RDA), which people can easily meet from their diets without supplements.

The RDA only stipulates the *minimum* amount of a nutrient required to prevent disease but says nothing about the *optimal* amount, counter the proponents. They maintain that supplements are safe within a broad range of intake and safety problems are rarely reported. They point to studies showing that people who take supplements are, in general, healthier.

The cited studies are flawed, claim detractors, because people who take supplements also tend to be more educated and have healthier lifestyles—two factors known to be correlated with good health. The health benefits of most supplements are unproven, they say, and products should not be allowed to be advertised as remedies for any particular disease unless there is some evidence that they work and do so safely.

The suggestion that supplements are not safe is *Alarmism* sugarcoating. Statistics show that supplements cause far less harm than FDA-approved prescription drugs.[192,193] This double standard has prompted some proponents to accuse western medicine of being a fascist regime bent on preserving its power by opposing all prevention of disease. Many supplements, they argue, have been used in other countries for centuries, long before the American Medical Association (AMA) nominated itself the world authority on treatment.

The argument is understandably contentious because billions of dollars of supplement product sales and quite possibly billions in medical and prescription fees are at stake.[194] Is it possible that both sides are right? Might there be some supplements that are proven effective by well-designed studies and others that are just pure wallet drainers? Yes, and you are about to learn how to tell the difference.

"If you have diabetes ..." reads the intriguing Internet news group posting, "exciting news is here." The post contains a link to a website where you can find out more about *The Greatest Vitamin in the World* and purchase a 30-day supply for about $50. Prominently displayed at the top of this web page is an offer for you to get paid $1000 every time you convince just twenty people to try these vitamins.

The $35 membership fee gets you your very own web "site" from which you will generate sales and earn thousands of dollars. Your "site" is actually just a web *page*, identical to the one you were directed to and every other page on the web site *dontforgettotakeyourvitamins.com*. There is one difference: your page is encoded with your unique "independent advertiser" number to keep track of your sales.

According to a CBS News consumer report, "independent advertiser" really means target of the operation.[195] The article uncovered how, shortly after a target's web page is online, she is baited with a few hits and sales, and then called by representatives selling expensive extras like "guaranteed traffic" and television ads that promise to bring more buyers to her web page. While her business flounders, she is given just enough hope that her site is on the verge of earning thousands in "residual income" if only she had the next traffic-enhancing product to get there. The "investment" ends up costing hundreds to thousands of dollars—however much can be taken from the target before she finally realizes that there is no hope and gives up.

While the scheme going on here may be somewhat obvious in hindsight, thanks to CBS News, most supplement sugarcoating is much more subtle. Sugarcoating is obscured by sophisticated schemes where product marketing is disguised as educational material that references scientific studies. The information is compelling and sometimes even true. Often products are endorsed by people in white coats, "certified" nutritionists, "doctors," "PhDs," and other pseudo health professionals who have obtained bogus credentials from unaccredited mail-order shops or simply made them up. This form of sugarcoating, called **Bullegitimacy**, is well documented in Stephen Barrett's expose, *The Vitamin Pushers: How the "Health Food" Industry is Selling America a Bill of Goods.*[196]

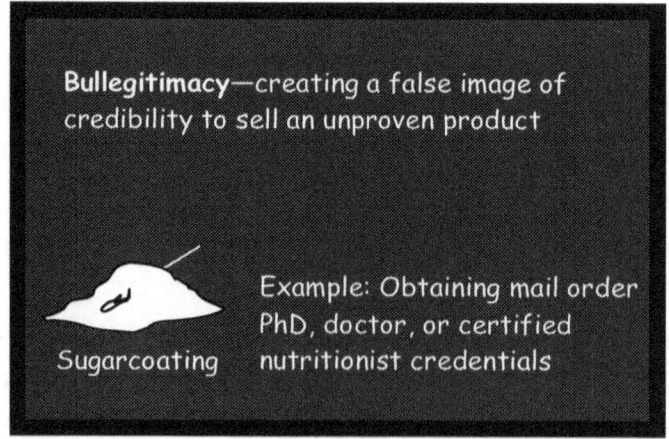

Chalkboard 7.1: Definition of Bullegitimacy

Since the days of snake oil, distributors of supplements and other remedies have known that the best way to move a product is to make health claims about it. Although it is illegal to put unproven health claims on a product label, the rules are so lenient that marketers have been able to make all kinds of claims by carefully wording their labels to avoid prosecution. For example, while it is illegal for a label to claim that a product "protects against heart disease" it can say that the product "promotes cardiovascular function" with little burden for proof. There are gaping loopholes for *Manufacting* in the regulation of supplement labels and essentially no regulation of other sources of information about the products. The desired message can be suggested with carefully constructed wording on the product label and then driven home explicitly through a variety of channels such as books, pamphlets, in-store lectures, advertisements, trade shows, newsletters, health expos, marketing literature, press conferences, PR agencies, chiropractors, naturopaths, nutrition consultants, physicians who practice "nutritional medicine," and others who are willing to make unfounded health claims.

Supplement manufacturers also use product labeling to create a false sense of security (*Guiltabsolution*). For example, supplements that are labeled "all natural," may not be. After the FDA received numerous reports of serious and life-threatening adverse events related to the supplement "Nature's Nutrition Formula One," investigations uncovered that, although the product was marketed as an all natural nutritional supplement made from plant ingredients, it was actually spiked with two pharmaceutical-grade chemicals, ephedrine hydrochloride and caffeine anhydrous. The manufacturer pleaded guilty to defrauding the United States government and misleading FDA investigators.[197,198]

Although the overwhelming majority of supplements are safe

to take at normal dosages, safety concerns are occasionally real. Over the decade from 1993 to 2003 the FDA received 5,574 reports of adverse events associated with dietary supplements.[199] Nearly half of those reports were associated with a supplement called Ephedra (a.k.a. ma huang). A naturally occurring substance derived from plants, Ephedra was marketed as a weight loss and sports performance aid, but it was also associated with heart attacks and strokes. In 2004, the FDA banned sales of dietary supplements containing ephedrine, the plant's active ingredient.

Whereas the natural plant source, Ma huang, has been used in China for thousands of years to treat various ailments, in the U.S. the active ingredient was extracted, concentrated into pill form, and swallowed like speed to induce weight loss. This type of use is far from traditional and at high dosages can be extremely harmful. The story of ephedra reminds us not to assume that just because a substance comes from a plant and has been used in eastern medicine for centuries it will be safe to take in pill form. Remember, alcohol, cocaine, and heroin are all substances derived from plants.

One of the most successfully marketed unproven health claims is the belief that B vitamins help us to deal with emotional stress. This impression was created and reinforced by completely unsubstantiated marketing slogans such as "Stress robs us of essential nutrients" and "A busy lifestyle puts extra demands on your body." The notion that high-dosage vitamins should be used to treat stress probably originates with the 1952 National Academy of Sciences report, *Therapeutic Nutrition*, which recommends vitamins for people suffering from serious *physical* stresses such as surgery, serious burns, or major fractures. There's no evidence that vitamins effectively treat *emotional* stress, a loosely defined condition that could apply to anyone. Nonetheless, ads for "stress formula" vitamins promote these vitamins as a targeted therapy — not to people who have burns, fractures, or surgery, but to people who feel busy or over-worked.

When cornered, supplement makers will insist that their ads are talking only about physical stress, though their marketing slogans clearly indicate otherwise.[200] In 1986 New York State forced the discontinuation of *Stresstabs* ads that implied that the vitamins were therapeutic for emotional stress.[201] By extending the rare circumstance of physical stress to the everyday one of emotional stress, marketers of stress supplements are employing *Overgeneralization* to expand their customer base. How many Americans think they are busy or have stress in their lives?

Among the most effective (and completely legal) ways of making unproven health claims is to disguise them as education. Have you ever wondered why health food stores always have little bookstores in them? Educational books, magazines, pamphlets, and websites — the silent sales force — are the primary marketing tools of health products. The multi-billon dollar supplement industry generates an enormous amount of product marketing in the form of health education materials. This is a form of sugarcoating called *Edumarketing*.

Consider *The Diabetes Cure*, a popular book co-authored by Dr. Vern Cherewatenko, general physician, and Paul Perry, professional writer. Although the use of the word *cure* in the title might create a hint of suspicion, at first glance nothing about the book seems out of the ordinary. However, the reader may not be aware that the authors have co-written another book, *The Stress Cure, A Simple 7-Step Plan to Balance Mood, Improve Memory, and Restore Energy*, which promotes the supplement DHEA and tells you how you can buy it from a supplement company called

HealthMax. Author Cherewatenko happens to be the president and CEO of HealthMax.

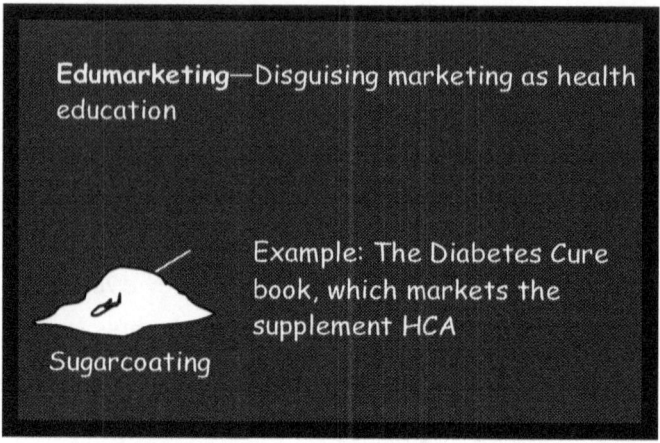

Chalkboard 7.2: Definition of Edumarketing

The cornerstone of Cherewatenko's cure for diabetes is supplementation with Hydroxy Citric Acid (HCA), which is also sold by HealthMax. In *The Diabetes Cure* Cherewatenko claims, "For a natural approach to curing most cases of type 2 diabetes, HCA cannot be beat." It seems truly amazing that Cherewatenko has found a cure for diabetes that has eluded the world's greatest research scientists. In his "Nine Steps to a Cure" chapter, Cherewatenko provides a four-page list of HCA products and where to get them, including vendor names, phone numbers and pricing. Second on the list is Dr. Cherewatenko's company, HealthMax, and at the top is I.D.E.A. Concepts of Englewood CO. Who is I.D.E.A Concepts I wondered.

Internet archives reveal that I.D.E.A Concepts was a multi-level marketing (MLM) network formed in 1995 to sell products such as *Vitamin O* liquid oxygen, *Instant Sparkle* tooth whitening sticks, the *Ultimate Wrinkle Care System*, and the *Ionic Laundryball* (based on "space age liquid micro magnet technology"). I.D.E.A. began advertising via email in 1996 with sales pitches for liquid oxygen and solicitations for "independent advertisers" who would sell I.D.E.A. products from personal web pages. (Does this sound familiar?)

What's the connection with Cherewatenko and his book? The answer can be found in the Internet newsgroup *misc.health.diabetes.*[202] On October 29, 1998 one of I.D.E.A. Concepts' independent advertisers, Nancy Kramer, posted the following message to the newsgroup:

```
IDEA Concepts, Inc., a health and wellness firm out of
Denver, Colorado, has just become affiliated with a
prominent M.D. who has written a major book to be
published soon by a major New York publishing firm,
Harper Collins.

...

The book is THE DIABETES CURE. The doctor is Dr. Vern
Cherewatenko, and the product he describes as central
to this medical approach to slowing, stopping, or
curing diabetes is available only through IDEA
Concepts. It's called Ultimate HCA with Chromium and
Vanadium. Let me tell you a bit more.

...

The product will be available in December. Dr. Vern
will be promoting it on talk shows nationwide very
soon; in fact, he had just gotten off the air after
doing his TalkAmerica radio show, aired in 400,000
cities worldwide, when I talked with him Tuesday night
on our National Conference Call.
```

The above are excerpts from a longer post, but they reveal the *Edumarketing* going on with *The Diabetes Cure*. The signature at the end of Kramer's posting was telling. It read:

```
Nancy Kramer
Lifestyle Specialist
I.D.E.A. Concepts, Inc. in association with HealthMax,
Incorporated
```

HealthMax, you may recall, is Dr. Cherewatenko's company, whose HCA product was listed second to I.D.E.A.'s.

Curious as to what a "Lifestyle Specialist" was, I "googled"

Ms. Kramer. When I checked in early 2006, Nancy was advertising a breast enhancement product on her very own web page, which said, "This Affiliate Site is Owned By Nancy Kramer, ID #103."[203] The product, *All Natural Curves*, was developed by I.D.E.A. Concepts founder Ken Hampshire and marketed under I.D.E.A.'s new moniker, Advanced Health Group.

Advanced Health Group still markets an HCA product for type 2 diabetes. With a new name and a new clinical, scientific image that includes pictures of people donning medical scrubs and white lab coats, Advanced Health Group now appears to be a sophisticated provider of alternative medicine that has disassociated itself from the multi-level marketing scheme that was I.D.E.A. Concepts (though, as of July 2006, the title of their nutritionals web page was still, "Welcome to IDEA Concepts").[204] I.D.E.A.'s founders appear to have learned that by appearing as a scientifically based health company, they are more likely to earn the trust of unsuspecting customers and sell more products.

"To secure an endorsement from healthcare professionals with the ultimate objective of getting its products adopted as a standard treatment for diabetes management" is the stated goal of pharmaceutical-turned-supplement maker Nutrition 21 Incorporated.[205] Nutrition 21 markets chromium supplements, which they claim improve insulin sensitivity. Chromium is a trace mineral that is thought to play a role in insulin action, though no one knows exactly how.

A key element of Nutrition 21's marketing strategy (according to the company's "About Us" web page) is to publicize the results of clinical trials supporting chromium. The company funds many of these trials and boasts to investors about its "research alliances with leading universities, research institutes and scientists."[206]

Several independent studies, however, did not find benefits to chromium supplementation and some have suggested safety problems.[207,208] In large-scale studies conducted in China and Finland, supplementation with large doses of chromium decreased glucose levels in type 2 diabetics; however, other studies performed in Tunisia, the US and Israel showed no effect.[209,210,211,212,213,214] These results suggest that chromium supplementation may only help those who are deficient and that Americans, Israelis, and Tunisians aren't. However, an alternative interpretation (one favored by Nutrition 21) is that the trials failed to show benefit because they used forms of chromium that were not as biologically available as chromium *picolinate.*

Chromium picolinate is a neutralized form of chromium that was developed and patented by Dr. Gary Evans and a team of researchers at the USDA. That patent has been exclusively licensed by Nutrition 21, who has also hired Evans as a consultant and spokesperson. Evans has written a book, *Chromium Picolinate*, praising the supplement's numerous purported health benefits. Printed boldly on the cover, which includes pictures of chiseled male and female models, are the following claims:

FOR FAT LOSS

FOR HYPOGLYCEMIA

FOR LOWER CHOLESTEROL

FOR MUSCLE MASS

FOR INSULIN CONTROL

FOR LONGER LIFE

Although the Federal Trade Commission has ordered Nutrition 21 to stop making unsubstantiated weight loss and health claims for chromium picolinate, the company can continue to do so through Evans' book without violating any regulations. *Edumarketing* is an effective way to get around regulation and make unapproved health claims.

Edumarketing of supplements has become rampant in recent years thanks to the supplement industry's highly successful efforts to weaken the laws regulating supplements. In 1993, a letter-writing campaign resulted in the passing of new laws giving supplement companies the freedom to make health claims on product labels without prior FDA approval. The new legislation established that literature distributed at the point of sale (*Edumarketing*) was not subject to labeling laws and shifted the burden for proving supplement safety from product manufacturers to the understaffed FDA. This has effectively placed the burden for investigating the efficacy of supplements on us, the consumers.

Now that we understand that the burden is on us and not the FDA, what can we do to avoid being sugarcoated?

First, look for obvious warning signs. Whenever you come across an independent advertiser, realize the advertiser is probably more focused on moving product and creating "residual income" than on improving your health. Be skeptical of anything he tells you, and remember that most of his specialized knowledge of supplements comes from *Edumarketing* materials.

The same goes for literature and sales assistance you get at your local health food store. While it probably won't kill you to try out a recommended product, basing health decisions on a salesperson might. Alarming studies have shown that most health store salespeople are quick to prescribe remedies for any ailment, including deadly diseases such as cancer and AIDS.[215] Not all salespeople are that irresponsible. However, because some are, we should maintain a healthy level of skepticism when in the health food store and seek qualified second opinions.

Be wary of the word *cure*; it is a sensational word used to grab attention and sell. As of 2006, there is no known cure for any type of diabetes. The odds that there exists a real cure that only a handful of people know about are very, very, very slim in this age where news about Jennifer Aniston's love life travels at the speed of light.

If you can, investigate the evidence by looking at published studies. You can find them on the Internet using Pubmed's free search engine at http://www.ncbi.nlm.nih.gov/entrez/query.fcgi. Most supplements have at least one study supporting their efficacy and safety. If not, then that's a big clue. Evaluate the quality of the studies. Did the result come from placebo-controlled clinical trials involving more than a handful of patients and lasting more than two weeks or did the authors just report that some people who took the supplement for a short while felt better? Have the results been duplicated or do all the positive studies come from the same research group? Were the studies published in reputable, peer-reviewed journals with a reputation for integrity or just some magazine?

Don't believe everything you read. Realize that nearly all printed information about supplements is created for the express purpose of marketing the product. Don't buy anything sold on late night infomercials, even if you can with three easy payments of just $19.99. Avoid "ground floor" opportunities to earn residual income running a supplement business out of your home.

Validate the credentials of people claiming to be doctors, PhDs, and certified health professionals. Make sure they received their degrees from accredited universities and not mail order houses or quack shops. Look at what else these so-called experts have done in their career. Do they have a history of publishing articles in peer-reviewed medical journals or do they write books promoting pills sold by their own supplement company?

Beware of slogans and mantras, such as B vitamins for stress, that get repeated so many times that, despite lack of evidence, they just get absorbed into our subconscious and become accepted as common knowledge.

Finally, realize that because this industry is so loosely regulated, many sensational health claims for supplements, especially those found in "educational" books, pamphlets, and magazines, are false. Not all are, however. Some health claims are supported by a great deal of evidence. It is up to us to distinguish time-tested remedies from snake oil. This isn't easy. Studies evaluating the use of supplements to improve diabetes control and prevent complications often provide mixed results. This is not surprising, given the variability in what study participants eat. Those whose diets have vitamin and mineral deficiencies may realize more improvement than those who eat more nutritional foods.

What constitutes nutrient deficiency really depends on the individual. Everyone is unique in his genetic makeup, diet, and metabolism. In these areas diabetics are, by definition, very different from what is considered normal. In fact, diabetic patients have been observed to be deficient in vitamin C, vitamin E, magnesium, calcium, copper, folate, and zinc.[216,217,218,219,220,221,222,223,224,225,226,227] Thus, it makes sense to be informed about the supplements that are available to us. Appendix B reviews the evidence (or lack thereof) for a number of supplements used to treat diabetes. Whether or not these supplements help will ultimately depend on many factors, including our unique physiology, diet, and other environmental circumstances.

Fortunately, we have glucometers to help us determine which supplements, if any, meet our individual needs. Use your meter to see whether taking a supplement has any noticeable effect — positive or negative. Talk to your doctor about your experimentation with supplements. If your doctor is not supportive, find another doctor who recognizes that different people have different needs and who encourages you to investigate better ways to take care of yourself. As with everything, *listen* to what your meter says. Don't let its objective voice be drowned out by the marketing buzz. Finally, remember that supplements should complement, not replace healthy eating.

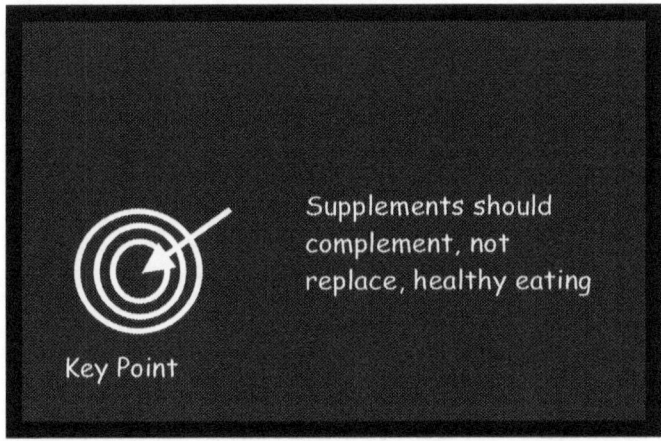

Chalkboard 7.3: Golden Rule for Supplements

Healthy eating is the subject of our next chapter: *The Principles of Eating Well.*

8

The Principles of Eating Well

In previous chapters we have seen how information about nutrition, supplements, and substitutes is replete with claims and theories that are based on marketing objectives, not facts. Now that we know the facts, we can discard the sugarcoating and put together an effective plan for healthy eating. Because each of us is unique, there is no one-size-fits-all dietary plan. Optimal nutrition requires a personalized approach. Thus, commandments such as "thou shalt limit thy intake of nutrient x to y percent of calories" serve no purpose. What will be useful is a set of general principles that guide us in our individual walk and recognize our diversity.

The Principles of Eating Well give us a great deal of freedom in making personal choices, but they also empower us to make the best ones. Because the principles are based on science without sugarcoating, there is no question or controversy; when you follow them you know you are eating the healthiest diet for managing your diabetes. Let these principles guide you in making daily choices.

Principle #1: Lose your intuition

Just as airplane pilots must train themselves to ignore their instincts and rely on their instruments when flying in sight-limited conditions, we must train ourselves to let go of any preconceived (sugarcoated) notions we have about diet and rely only on the facts before us. Our intuition does not serve us because it is built upon sugarcoated marketing messages that have deeply penetrated our consciousness. For example, logically you know the facts about essential fatty acids and realize the foolishness of blaming health problems on a single nutrient, yet you still *feel* it would be prudent to use low fat versions of foods. Let go of such attachments; they will undermine your efforts to succeed because they contradict the science. Following them is not an insurance policy, but rather a way to fatten up and increase your risk for heart disease.

Sugarcoated marketing has instilled in us several erroneous pre-conceived notions—about nutrition bars, sugar-free junk food, chromium supplements, etc. Forget them and pay close attention to your glucometer and the nutrition facts on product labels. The facts will often surprise you and this will help rid you of preconceived notions. When you look at labels you'll see that low fat versions of products are missing more "good" fats than "bad." Many have added carbohydrates. You'll realize that "sugar-free" products still contain high amounts of carbohydrates and do, in fact, have a "net impact" on blood sugar. You may be surprised that an 8oz container of low fat, fruit-added yogurt has twice the sugar of a regular sized bag of peanut M&M's.

Nonfat yogurt is a classic example of a junk food that many Americans intuitively feel is healthy because it contains no fat. Our intuition leads us to believe we have license to consume copious amounts of this "free" food. Buying into the "pleasure without guilt" promise (*Guiltabsolution*) of nonfat frozen yogurt, Americans fattened up because we didn't follow principle number two.

Principle #2: Focus on grams of *food*

Our obsession with cutting back on a single nutrient to some percentage of calories has blinded us to the more important factor—the *absolute number* of calories we are consuming. One easy and effective way to reduce the percentage of calories from fat in your diet is to gorge yourself on rice cakes and fat-free frozen yogurt. The more carbohydrates you consume, the lower the percentage of fat becomes. This is how Americans got fat in the low fat era; while the *percentage* of dietary fat decreased, *overall* caloric intake (including calories from fat) increased along with the incidence of obesity. Nowadays, many of us have reversed direction by cutting carbs and eating more protein and fat, but if we don't cut down on calories we will continue to get fatter.

Our problem is not too many grams of fat or too many grams of carbs; it is all of the above. As we have seen, there is no evil nutrient, which, when eliminated from the diet, will deliver us to weight loss and healthiness. The solution is not sugar-free ice cream or fat-free cookies; it is simply to eat less. We are overweight and unhealthy because we eat too much. Rather than worry about the number of grams of fat or grams of carbohydrate in a serving, let's focus on the number of grams *on the plate*. It's easier to measure and a better indicator of how fat the meal is going to make us. One of the most powerful ways to reduce grams of food is principle number three.

Principle #3: Snack Frequently

If you pay attention to your glucometer, you've probably

noticed that blood sugar spikes often occur after big meals. There are numerous methods for flattening out these spikes, the best being to simply *consume less* at mealtime. A great way to do this without feeling deprived or hungry is by snacking.

If there's anything sexy about a fact-based, healthy diet it's that we get to spoil our appetites. Overeating is common when a big plate of delicious food is placed in front of a very hungry person because there is a significant time lag between eating enough and feeling full. During this lag it's easy to pack in plenty of excess calories, especially when you're hungry. The solution is to get the clock started early by eating a small snack before you eat your meal.

Many of us have witnessed the effectiveness of bread service at spoiling an appetite. While this works, there are more efficient and nutritious choices that won't raise your blood sugar as much as white bread. Foods containing protein and fiber generally lead to a greater feeling of fullness.[228] A salad containing some amount of protein (e.g., spinach, beans, hard boiled eggs, or cheese) is a wonderfully nutritious way to spoil your appetite. Edamame (soy beans) and nuts are naturally high in protein and fiber and make excellent pre-meal snacks. Mixed nuts are great anytime snacks because they are nutritious and convenient to carry around. Not only will snacking keep your metabolism up and help you to feel full sooner, it will add variety to your diet, which is necessary for getting the full range of nutrients that your body needs. This brings us to principle number four.

Principle #4: Eat real food

It is certainly possible to get all of the fifty or so known essential nutrients from a diet of nutrition bars, shakes, and vitamin pills. However, supplements and supplement-fortified foods are poor substitutes for real food sources of nutrients. Food naturally contains many more substances whose functions in our bodies are not yet fully understood. Our bodies depend on the entire package of nutrients, not just the ones listed on the Centrum label.

Whole foods that haven't been stripped of nutrients, e.g., whole grains, fruits, vegetables, and meat are preferable to foods like white bread, breakfast cereal, and nutrition bars, which are fortified with spray-on nutrients. A good litmus test for whole foods is to ask the question: when was this food invented? The longer ago the better. Foods with the highest density of nutrients—fruits, vegetables, whole grains, nuts, seeds, legumes, and meat—have all been a part of the human diet for millennia. On the other hand, take a look at a sampling of what the last two centuries of food innovation have brought us:

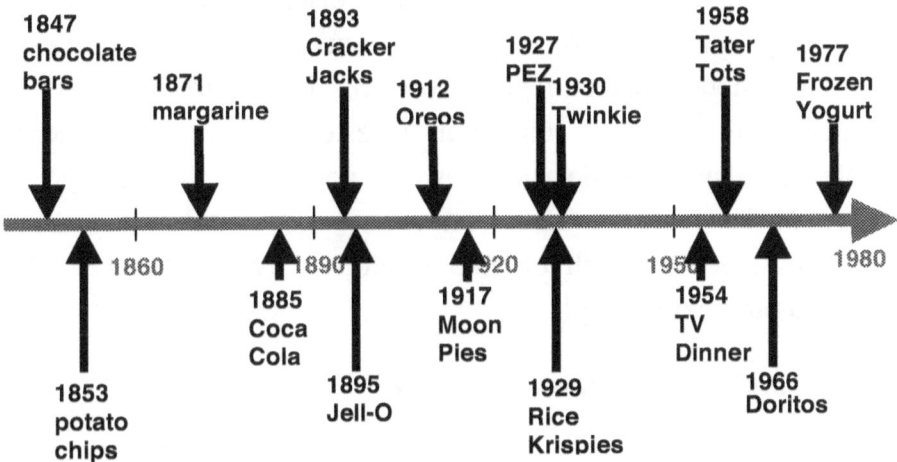

Figure 8.1: A timeline of recent advances in food technology

Invention in the modern era doesn't *cause* a food to be unhealthy, there just happens to be a very strong *correlation*. This may be because our bodies have not yet adapted to cope with modern inventions that have improved the efficiency of producing and distributing food. On the evolutionary time scale, the invention of flour is a relatively recent one. Even more recently, sugar refinement and the invention of high fructose corn syrup have made it possible to compress a large number of calories into a small amount of food. Modern methods of hydrogenating vegetable oils to give baked goods a longer shelf life have created unnaturally high levels of harmful type of fat. Combine these three advances and you get modern miracles of food science such as the Twinkie. Perhaps several thousand years from now our metabolic systems will have evolved to survive on Twinkies and soda, but for now we are not well equipped to handle them.

As modern foods have been introduced to the U.S. over the last century, the per capita consumption of calories, and the incidence of obesity, diabetes, and heart disease have risen. We are not only consuming more calories, but we are burning fewer because modern technological advances have allowed us to be much more sedentary than our ancestors. Maintaining energy balance is much easier to do when you are active and prefer nutrient-rich foods that have been around for thousands of years to modern inventions full of empty calories. This is the key idea behind our next principle.

Principle #5: Succeed with HELP

Yes, you *can* eat anything you want … as long as you (1) get all your essential nutrients and (2) don't eat too many calories. These two stipulations make up the principle of HELP: *High Essentials / Lighter Portions.* HELP is about getting more "bang for the buck" from the foods we eat by choosing foods that are highest in essentials (the vitamins, minerals, fatty acids, and amino acids that our body needs) and keeping portion sizes reasonable.

In America, diets are concerned with deprivation: what to cut out instead of what to eat. Under HELP, we are not concerned with limiting the percentage of calories from any particular nutrient, but with maximizing the amount of nutrition we get from each calorie. HELP naturally limits carbohydrates and undesirable types of fat because, being non-essential nutrients, they only serve to add calories and decrease the nutrition per calorie in a food. For example, a chocolate and candy covered peanut contains all the essentials of a regular peanut, but because it adds sugar and non-essential fats it has fewer essentials per calorie. Under the HELP principle, we would keep portions of both low, but prefer peanuts to chocolate candy peanuts to get more essentials per calorie.

It's easy to gain weight on a diet of empty calorie foods. Getting all the nutrients your body needs without gaining weight requires that you eat primarily nutrient-dense foods like vegetables, meat, and fish. Following the HELP principle will ensure that while your diet includes any food your heart desires it will always be predominantly made up of nutrient rich foods. A more detailed explanation of nutrient density and a full description of the HELP principle are given in Appendix D.

Unlike some popular diets, HELP comes with no "eat all you want" promise. There is no gimmick; you just have to eat less junk food, more nutritious food, and smaller portions. I'm sorry, there aren't any chocolate bars or shakes that come with this diet. HELP may not be as sexy as the latest fad diet but it has a unique advantage: it is based on facts, not sugarcoating, so it works. Don't just take my word for it; test it out with principle number six.

Principle #6: Trust your meter

One thing you can always trust is your meter. When properly calibrated, your glucometer provides the most accurate, personal, unbiased, and valuable information you will find. Tap into its power.

One of the most powerful things you can do with your meter is determine precisely how a mixed meal will affect your blood sugar. One of the biggest drawbacks of using the glycemic load as a prediction tool is that the experiments used to determine the numbers weren't performed on you. Moreover, glycemic load numbers only apply to a single serving of a specific type of food, but meals consist of several foods, which are not always served in standard serving sizes. Even if you go through the trouble of estimating portion sizes, consulting tables, and performing calculations to come up with a rough approximation, you still have the problem that that different foods affect each other's glycemic load when they are mixed together.

Rather than bother with all that, why not just *measure* your personal glycemic response to the entire meal? Determining the personal glycemic response is easy, and best of all, the measurements are all performed on you, so they directly apply to you. A glucometer and five test strips is all it takes. Here's how it works:

Step 1: Prepare the meal of your choice

Step 2: Measure your blood sugar right before you begin eating. Then eat as much as you normally would.

Step 3: Measure your blood sugar thirty minutes after you took your first bite. Subtract the pre-meal value and write this number down. For example, if your blood sugar was 90 before you began eating and it is now 146, write down 56.

Step 4: Repeat step 3 at one hour, ninety minutes, and two hours

Step 5: Add the four numbers your wrote down together and then divide them by four. This is your personal glycemic response. As with the glycemic load, the lower the number the better.

```
Personal Glycemic Response

Time          BG        difference
0             90        -
30 min        146       56
1 hour        178       88
90 min        152       62
2 hour        132       42
--------------------------------------
total                  248 / 4   62

personal glycemic response = 62
```

Chalkboard 8.1: Calculating Personal Glycemic Response

Personal glycemic response values are computed differently than glycemic load or glycemic index values, so it makes no sense to compare them. Whereas the glycemic index and glycemic load deal with measurements of how single foods affected other people, the personal glycemic response indicates how mixed meals affect you, with no calculations required.

The more times you repeat this experiment on a meal the better idea you will have of how it affects you. The results will be more consistent if you have the meal prepared the same way and eat the same amount each time. Taking medication, especially insulin, may add some variability to the numbers, but this variability is useful information. If you change your medication regime, comparing data recorded before the change to data recorded after the change will help you to see the effect of the medication change.

Being able to predict how your body will respond to various meals and changes in medication are important benefits of knowing your personal glycemic response. The personal glycemic response is exactly the kind of information we need to make optimal choices for our health. There's currently no better tool for managing diabetes than your glucometer.

Principle #7: Avoid culture traps

Perhaps the biggest health problem facing Americans is our own culture. In the United States food is so abundant that it is used as a form of entertainment, like going for ice cream, making brownies, or getting pizza. It doesn't matter what time of day or how hungry we are, because these are not meals but social events. At work we socialize over donuts and pastries. At school we find candy, cookies, and soda in the vending machine. At birthday parties we pass around the cake and soda. At the movies popcorn, candy, and soda are an integral part of the experience. At the game, the concert, the beach, the zoo, the amusement park, and any event you can think of it's our tradition to consume hot dogs, ice cream, candy, chips, and, of course, more soda.

The use of food as entertainment exemplifies our culture of consumerism driven by marketing. In newspapers, magazines, television, radio, and the Internet we are bombarded with marketing messages to consume more and we do. American restaurants have successfully "super-sized" us. Nowadays it is almost unheard of to be served a normal sized portion of food (let alone a USDA sized portion) at a restaurant. Most restaurants serve huge portions that come with enough bread to feed your extended family for days.

Exacerbating the problem is our lack of movement. Television watching has become a national pastime, and remote controls allow us to watch more without ever having to leave the couch. We Americans live in a world of convenience, with automatic appliances, food processors, ride-on lawnmowers, clap-on lights, electronic can openers, automatic toilet flushers, motion-activated towel dispensers, and automobiles that take us effortlessly to places where elevators, escalators, automatic doors, and moving walkways ensure that we never have to burn an extra calorie.

A lifetime of inactivity and regular, empty-calorie social events makes us overweight and diabetic. We address the problem not by changing our ways, but with "healthy alternatives" such as Diet Coke, low-fat Pop-Tarts, and Atkins Advantage™ Bars. Like smokers who switch to light cigarettes, we maintain our cultural norms with a clear conscience, just as the manufacturer had hoped when they marketed the healthy perception to us. Just as tobacco manufacturers provide a multitude of different low tar and low nicotine products to choose from, junk food manufacturers offer us a plethora of low fat, fat-free, low carb, and sugar-free options. They spend billions of marketing dollars annually to convince us that these modified junk foods are healthy.

As Americans it is our unalienable right to eat all the junk food we want as long as it has an Atkins or AHA seal of approval. We see no need to stop consuming the products that define this great, fast food nation. After all, we've been told they're healthy and if anything goes wrong we can turn to our healthcare system. We have drugs to fix any problem that afflicts us and health insurance will cover the costs.

Adopting this typical American mentality will make you a typical American statistic. You will have a better than even chance of being overweight and you are far more likely to die from heart disease or the complications of diabetes than most other people on this planet. On the other hand, you have the power to change the odds, but this requires shedding a number of cultural norms. I have enumerated a few and you will have no trouble identifying them all if you just pay attention to what junk foods present themselves in various social situations. You already know what you should do; the real question is whether you are going to exercise discipline in making daily choices. Is eating that piece of cake really worth losing your eyesight? Pizza for a limb? Chocolate for a kidney?

Continually resisting cultural pressure is not easy, but it can be done and it is well worth the effort. Millions of Americans have made a personal commitment to their health. They skip the donuts, pass on the birthday cake, cut out the soda, and avoid fast food. They don't kid themselves about sugar-free junk food. They make the time to exercise instead of making excuses. These people are not statistics. They don't *hope* that they will live long, healthy, happy lives; they *know* they will. Their future is not up to chance. It is in their own hands, not in those of their healthcare provider, drug-maker, insurance company, or government.

When you put your health in the hands of these organizations, you are placing your trust in a system that pays lip service to diet and exercise but strongly emphasizes drug therapy. Despite the studies showing that lifestyle changes are more powerful than drugs, there is still a strong emphasis on prescription medication among American physicians.[229,230,231] Selling prescription drugs has become big business and the marketing practices now employed by pharmaceutical companies are far-reaching and highly effective. How drug companies sugarcoat our doctors and us is described in the third part of this book, Drugs.

Part III: Drugs

Throughout history, man has experimented with a variety of treatments for type 2 diabetes. The Chinese prescribed avoidance of sex and wine. The Egyptians recommended a diet of grains, fruit, and sweet beer. In ancient Greece, bloodletting and dehydration were the treatment of the day. Today we treat diabetes with a lifetime of pills and/or injections. Although we know vastly more about type 2 diabetes than our ancestors, we are not much better off; we still don't have a cure or even a treatment that prevents complications.

Not too long ago there were competing theories about the root cause of diabetes. Many scientists, noting the sweetness of diabetic urine, postulated that diabetes was caused by a defect of the kidney while a few others challenged the prevailing wisdom and suspected the pancreas. The matter was "settled" in 1850 by one of the most prominent and respected physiologists of the time, Claude Bernard. Bernard performed an experiment in which he sealed the pancreatic ducts of dogs to see if they would develop diabetes. The dogs did not, leading Bernard and other scientists to rule out the pancreas.

Of course we now know that they were wrong. What Bernard and colleagues didn't know at the time was that insulin (which wouldn't be discovered for another seventy years) is secreted through ductless glands, so plugging pancreatic ducts would have no effect on it whatsoever. It is easy to see in hindsight how Bernard, a brilliant scientist who made fundamental advancements in our understanding of diabetes, could employ rigorous scientific methods and logic only to reach an erroneous conclusion: *he didn't know what he didn't know.* Bernard's experiment reminds us that even the most logical conclusions of today's greatest minds may someday be overturned in light of new evidence. For incomplete knowledge is not just a phenomenon of the past. The present, like every moment of scientific history, is full of erroneous theories waiting to be proven false at some later time by someone with better information. Surely the future will hold as many epiphanies as the past, disproving or clarifying many of the theories we hold today.

The humble appreciation for what we don't know seems absent in the practice of modern western medicine. There is a disturbing confidence and frightening certainty that the medical treatment *du jour*, prescription drugs, is *the way* to treat everything, including diabetes. The makers of diabetes drugs don't have a cure for diabetes but we are expected to trust that, with all their cutting-edge technology, they have developed something much better than modern day bloodletting. We do trust them, much as our ancestors did their healers, because we trust science, which has brought the world useful things, like penicillin, electricity, and the cotton gin. Yet, despite all our medications, diabetes is still the leading cause of kidney failure, adult blindness, and non-traumatic amputation, and is the sixth leading cause of death in the United States.

The pharmaceutical industry spends extravagantly to draw focus away from the dismal reality of type 2 diabetes medications and to convince doctors and patients that these drugs are worth the high price tag they carry. However, the unspoken reality is that the medications currently used to treat type 2 diabetes do not provide lasting control of blood sugar or prevent complications. If this surprises you, then take the time to carefully examine the evidence you are about to see. It comes from the largest and longest clinical trials ever performed with type 2 medications and clearly shows the ineffectiveness of these drugs. Nonetheless, these very results have been sugarcoated to promote the sale of drugs and a false hope that they will make us better. This sugarcoating has resulted in financial hardship, physical suffering, and even the death of patients. The following chapters reveal the ways in which information about diabetes drugs is sugarcoated and tell the true story of how the consequences are sometimes deadly.

9

The Effectiveness of Diabetes Drugs

Thanks to prescription drugs, infectious diseases that were common and deadly only a few generations back are now rare and mostly treatable. Medicines are now used to successfully treat nearly every kind of medical condition from acid reflux to yeast infection. The power of an aspirin to relieve a headache or an antibiotic to clear up an infection in a few days is truly a miracle that we often take for granted. Because medicine has become so advanced and ubiquitous, we have come to expect that for every condition there will be a drug to clear it up.

I truly wish we had a pill that could clear up type 2 diabetes. Imagine a scenario in which you go to the doctor and are diagnosed with diabetes. Your doctor prescribes a pill that you take twice daily for seven days. At your follow-up visit, tests reveal that the condition is completely gone. You celebrate with a banana split and watch your blood glucose stay wonderfully normal. Of course, you wouldn't actually *watch* it because there would be no reason for you to own a glucometer and strips. You would just know that, thanks to the medicine, your insulin function was working perfectly normally again.

Unfortunately, we don't have that pill. Instead, what we have are drugs that must be taken every day for the rest of your life. These drugs are not designed to fix your metabolism, but to compensate for it in one of three ways:

- increase insulin (with insulin and sulfonylureas),
- improve insulin sensitivity (with metformin and TZDs)
- reduce the need for insulin (with starch blockers)

The above is a vastly simplified overview of diabetes medication, but will suffice for our purposes here (Appendix C provides a detailed, factual explanation of diabetes drugs and their safety and efficacy). For now, we need only understand that all of these drugs are based on the same theory, the Diabetes Drug Hypothesis, which states that taking diabetes drugs will lower blood glucose and prevent complications.

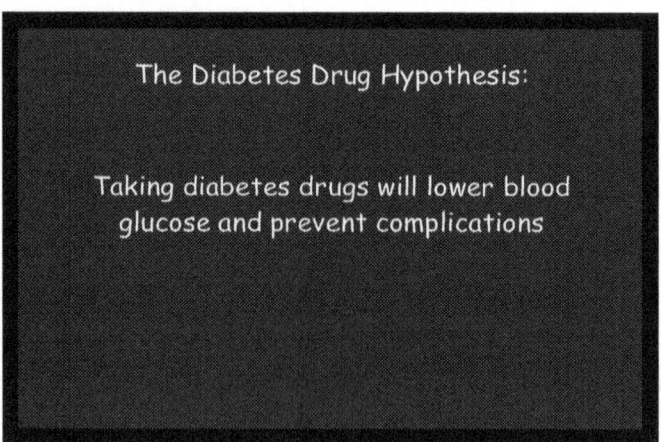

The Diabetes Drug Hypothesis:

Taking diabetes drugs will lower blood glucose and prevent complications

Chalkboard 9.1: The Diabetes Drug Hypothesis

This is a nice theory and if it were true, if diabetes drugs could prevent complications, then they might be worth the risks and costs associated with taking them. The unfortunate fact is, however, that many diabetic patients who diligently take their medications will suffer and die from the complications of diabetes anyway. After a lifetime of compliance and co-payments, there is no guarantee that you will be free of complications; there is only a *hope* that your chances of avoiding complications will be better.

The critical question is then *how much better*. To what degree will diabetes drugs improve my chances of avoiding complications?

The evidence necessary to answer this question comes from clinical trials that have carefully tracked large numbers of patients over several years to see which ones get complications and which ones don't. Such studies are rare since they require great amounts of time and resources, but fortunately, a few have been carried out. Each study monitored large groups of patients receiving either conventional therapy or intensive therapy (the exact definitions of these depend on the trial) and compared the outcomes of the groups over several years.

Two clinical trials, the Diabetes Control and Complications Trial and Stockholm Diabetes Intervention Study, followed patients with type 1 diabetes. In these studies all patients received insulin therapy, but patients in the intensive group monitored their blood sugar more frequently, injected insulin more frequently, visited the clinic more frequently, and had greater access to their healthcare team. In both studies, patients in the intensive group had lower HbA1c scores and fewer complications.[232,233] This evidence suggests that, for type 1 patients, paying more attention to your diabetes will help prevent complications. However, because all study participants took insulin, these studies do not address our question. To show how much better drug therapy is than non-drug therapy we need a study that compares the two.

Thus far, there have been two large-scale randomized clinical trials that have compared drug therapy to non-drug therapy for patients with type 2 diabetes. The first study, The University Group Diabetes Program (UGDP), tracked over a thousand patients throughout the 1960s and 1970s. The UGDP compared a conventional group, taking placebo, to four different intensive treatment groups (two types of insulin therapy and two different oral medications) to see which types of treatments worked best. None of the groups fared any better than the others, but the investigators did find that patients treated with the oral medications (tolbutamide and phenformin) were two and a half times as likely to die of a heart attack than those taking placebo.[234,235] Due to this result, both of the oral medication arms of the study were discontinued on ethical grounds.

Although the UGDP was a landmark trial for its time, its findings were harshly criticized.[236] Many asserted that the UGDP did not answer the question whether drug therapy prevents complications. The UGDP certainly did not provide the support for the Diabetes Drug Hypothesis many were seeking.

That support would come (ironically, as we shall see) from the United Kingdom Prospective Diabetes Study (UKPDS), which tracked type 2 diabetic patients through the 1980s and 1990s. This study compared a conventional therapy of diet education (with no drugs) to four types of intensive therapies: insulin and three different oral medications. At the study's outset, researchers had expected to see a 40% reduction in complications in the intensive therapy patients, but it soon became clear that that was not going to happen. After ten years, there was *no difference* in outcomes between the drug and non-drug treatment groups. UKPDS investigators admitted, "by 1987 no risk reduction was seen in any of these [outcomes] and it became obvious a 40% advantage was unlikely to be obtained."[237]

Nonetheless, the study carried on, in search of evidence that would support the Diabetes Drug Hypothesis. The problem, as the data from the UKPDS showed, was two-fold. First, the drugs didn't provide the "intensive blood glucose control" that was expected. All treatments in the UKPDS failed to keep blood sugar, (as measured by median HbA1c) in the normal range beyond one year. Figure 9.1 shows the median HbA1c levels of the drug and non-drug groups over fifteen years of study. The flat line at the bottom of the graph indicates the intensive blood glucose control that the study designers had hoped for when setting the goals for the drug treatment groups. As is clear from the data, none of the drug therapies even came close.

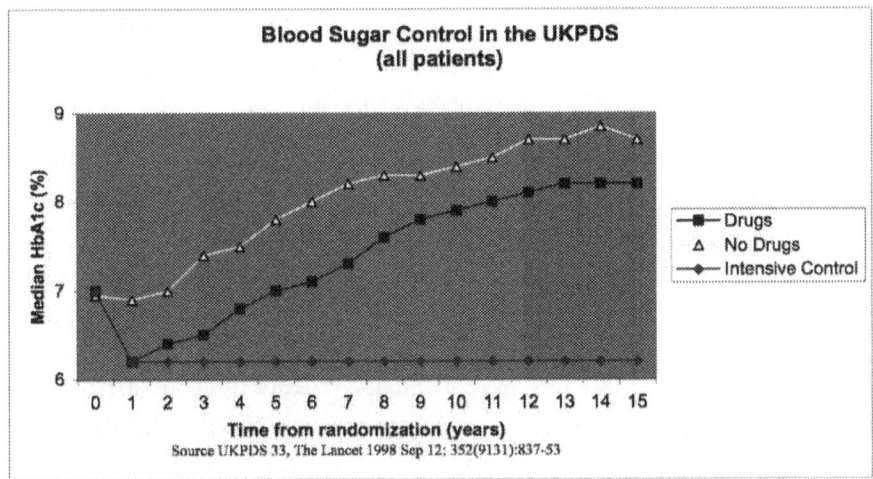

Figure 9.1 Blood sugar control of drug and diet groups in the UKPDS

The second problem was that the drugs didn't prevent any serious complications of diabetes. Over fifteen years of treatment, there were *no differences* in macrovascular complications (e.g. heart attack and stroke) or major microvascular complications (e.g. blindness, kidney failure, and amputation).[238] Whereas the study investigators admitted observing no differences in macrovascular complications, they curiously wrote, "Intensive blood-glucose control by either sulphonylureas or insulin substantially decreases the risk of microvascular complications."[239] This conclusion seems a bit strong, given that all complications occurred at similar rates in drug and non-drug groups (see Figure 9.2) with just *one* statistically significant exception: the need for retinal photocoagulation occurred in 10.3 percent of patients in the non-drug but only 7.6 percent in the drug group.

Retinal photocoagulation is a medical procedure that uses a laser to seal the eye's retina and stop vessels from growing and leaking. The need for this procedure is not a complication per se, but an *indicator* of progression toward blindness as determined by the opinion of a physician. This indicator, admitted the authors, accounted for the majority of the difference in microvascular disease between drug and non-drug treated patients. You might say that it accounted for *all* the difference; after fifteen years, researchers observed no statistically significant differences in any outcome except this one indicator (Figure 9.2).

What about the complication indicated by the indicator? According to the UKPDS investigators, "there was no difference between conventional and intensive treatments in the deterioration of visual acuity."[240] Nonetheless, combining all microvascular outcomes together (*Obfuscation*) allowed the UKPDS investigators to conclude that using drugs "substantially decreases the risk of microvascular complications." Such *Obfuscation* allows one to make broad and misleading statements that imply that drugs prevent blindness, kidney failure, and amputations even though, as the UKPDS data showed, they don't.

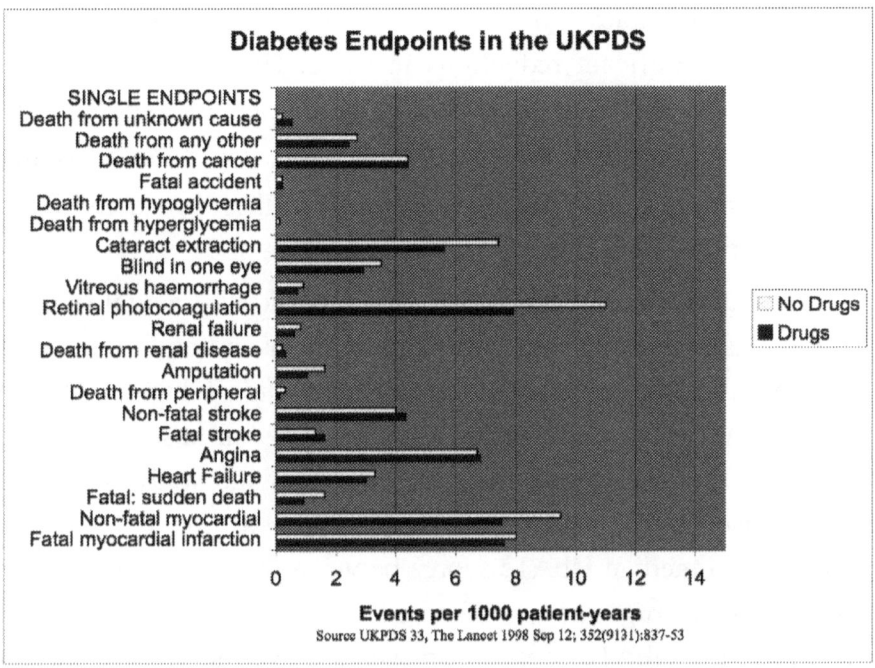

Figure 9.2 Comparison of complications in drug and non-drug groups in the UKPDS

The American Diabetes Association interpreted the UKPDS results as follows: "a significant reduction in complications was achieved with intensive therapy that lowered HbAlc levels to a median of 7.0% over 10 years when compared with conventional treatment that achieved a median HbAlc of 7.9%."[241]

Now this is an interpretation that needs interpretation. First, the word "significant" doesn't mean "significant," as in considerable or substantial, it's just shorthand for *statistically* significant. It applies to a rather small reduction (2.7 percent) in a single indicator (the need for retinal photocoagulation). *Glorification* turns a small difference in one indicator into a "significant reduction in complications." Moreover, the word "complications" doesn't mean blindness, amputation, kidney failure, heart attack, or stroke because there weren't any statistically significant reductions in these. Here "complications" means the need for retinal photocoagulation. As we've seen, *Obfuscation* extends this one indicator to "microvascular complications" and *Overgeneralization* further broadens it to "complications."

The ADA's use of the word "lowered" doesn't actually mean *lowered*, as in starting out with some number and ending up with some number that is lower, because that didn't happen in the UKPDS. As we saw in Figure 9.1, there was an absolute *rise* in HbA1c in the drug group over the course of the study. Here the ADA's use of the word "lowered" refers to the 0.9 percent *difference* in median HbA1c scores between the drug-taking group and the non-drug group observed over the first ten years. Strangely, the HbA1c scores from years eleven to fifteen are not included in this figure even though most of the "significant" difference in outcomes (well, one outcome actually) was observed during those years (see Figure 9.3). In years eleven to fifteen the median HbA1c in the drug group rose above 8.0 percent and the difference between drug and non-drug groups contracted to just 0.6 percent (Figure 9.1).[242] Using outcome data from years eleven to fifteen while ignoring the corresponding HbA1c data is a classic example of *Selective Omission*.

It is not surprising that this kind of HbA1c "lowering" did not prevent any major complications, as the Diabetes Drug Hypothesis would predict. Nonetheless, the ADA asserts that the "significant reduction in complications" was due to the "lowering" of HbA1c using drugs—i.e., the Diabetes Drug Hypothesis exactly. This direct contradiction of the study results, which showed no benefit of drugs on twenty out of twenty-one outcomes, appears to be a case of *Sponsorship*. The ADA's interpretation reflects exactly what pharmaceutical companies, who sponsor the ADA, want you, your doctor, and diabetes educator to believe: that diabetes drugs will lower your blood glucose and prevent complications.

In the UKPDS the likelihood of complications increased as patients' HbA1c scores went up, whether or not they took drugs (Figure 9.3). Nonetheless, the study investigators elected to phrase this observation in terms of HbA1c *lowering*, as, "Each 1% reduction in updated mean HbA1c was associated with reductions in risk of [...] 37% for microvascular complications."[243] (Note the *Mislinearization*; the "trend" is derived from only one data point). More accurately, the investigators could have said, "Each 1% *increase* in HbA1c *increases* the risk of microvascular complications by 69%," because that's what actually happened— HbA1c scores *increased* over time for people on drugs as did the incidence of microvascular complications (Figures 9.1 and 9.3). This choice of phrasing, however, doesn't give patients or doctors a warm fuzzy feeling about efficacy of diabetes drugs.

The data shown in Figure 9.3 objectively answers our question of how much better drugs are at preventing complications. The graph shows how drug therapy fared against non-drug therapy in preventing all diabetic complications in the UKPDS. Each individual plot shows the percentage of patients in a specific treatment group that experienced complications over fifteen years of monitoring. In addition to the actual data for the drug and non-drug groups, there is a third plot of the curve that one might expect to see for a more effective therapy that significantly reduced the frequency of diabetic complications. This is the sort of plot that the study designers had anticipated for drug therapy, but what they observed was a plot nearly identical to that seen in the non-drug therapy group.

Thus the answer our question is clear: both major type 2 clinical trials found drug therapy to be slightly to no better at preventing complications than non-drug therapy. Only through the liberal use of *Glorification, Obfuscation, Overgeneralization, Selective Omission,* and *Sponsorship* do we arrive at the perception that drugs are much more effective.

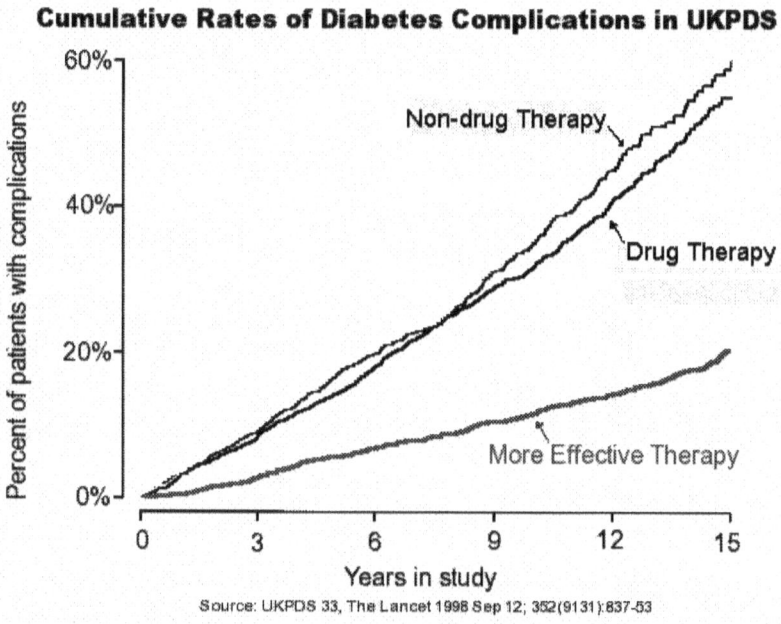

Figure 9.3: Comparison of complications in drug and non-drug groups in the UKPDS

It is possible that the one statistically significant difference observed in the UKPDS, the need for retinal photocoagulation, was entirely due to chance. By definition, the probability of obtaining a statistically significant result by chance is very small—like hitting a long shot at the race track—but, as everyone knows, the more often you play, the more likely you are to hit. In the UKPDS, where twenty-one different outcomes were measured and a ninety-nine percent confidence interval was used, the probability of observing at least one statistically significant outcome by chance was about one in five.

In fact, the "extremes of the play of chance" was suggested by investigators as an explanation for an unpleasant result that occurred in a UKPDS sub-study involving the drug metformin.[244] In this sub-study, which compared the outcomes of 342 obese patients treated with metformin to those of 411 obese patients receiving only diet education, a statistically significant *ninety-six percent increase* in risk of diabetes-related death occurred when metformin was added to another oral medication. As in the main study, there was an initial drop in HbA1c in the first year, but it then rose in both groups, year after year, reaching a median of 8.0 in the non-drug group and 7.4 in the metformin group over ten years (8.8 versus 8.3 in years eleven to fifteen). The interesting result is that while metformin didn't "lower" HbA1c as much as the drugs in the main UKPDS study it did produce a statistically significant reduction in heart attacks — something the other drug therapies did not do. This result suggests that there may be some benefit to metformin other than glucose "lowering." Figure 9.4 shows the frequency with which complications occurred in the metformin and non-drug therapy groups in the UKPDS sub-study. Like the other oral medications studied in the UKPDS, metformin therapy is slightly to no better at preventing microvascular complications than non-drug therapy.

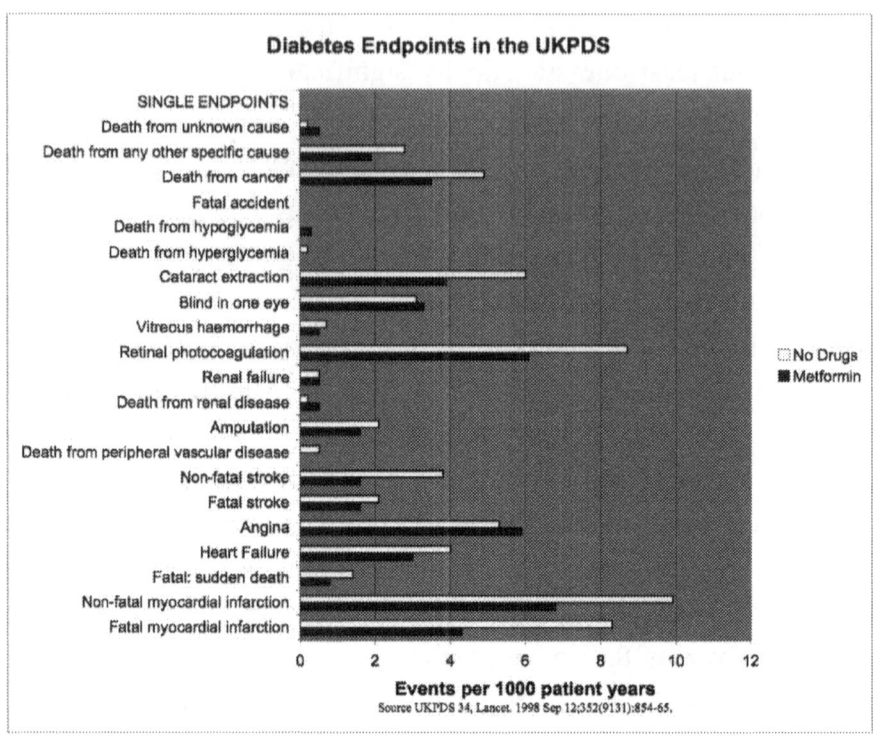

Figure 9.4 Comparison of complications in Metformin and no drug groups.

There are two important classes of diabetes medications not studied in the UKPDS. The "Carbinators" (alpha-glucosidase inhibitors) and TZDs (thiazolidinediones) have been shown to lower HbA1c in clinical trials.[245,246,247,248,249,250,251,252,253,254,255] By "lower" I mean just that; at the end of the study patients taking the drugs had lower HbA1c scores than when they started. However, the catch is that these trials didn't last very long—a year at most—making it easy to demonstrate glucose lowering. UKPDS data suggest that HbA1c lowering is a short-term effect that occurs in the first year after drug therapy is initiated.[256] Whether Carbinators or TZDs will provide lowering of blood glucose beyond one year or prevent complications is unknown, as no evidence that they do so currently exists. None of the studies with these drugs have lasted long enough to measure complications, which can take many years to occur.

Presently, there are at least three long-term clinical trials that are looking at the relationship of TZD therapy to outcomes. The PROACTIVE and RECORD studies are evaluating whether cardiovascular outcomes in people with type 2 diabetes can be prevented by pioglitazone (marketed as Actos) and rosiglitazone (marketed as Avandia) respectively and the DREAM trial is investigating whether rosiglitazone can prevent diabetes and atherosclerosis in pre-diabetic patients.[257,258,259] These trials should give us more insight into the long-term effectiveness of these new drugs.

The sum of evidence thus far indicates that diabetes drugs provide a short-term glucose lowering benefit that does not make a significant (i.e., considerable or substantial) difference in preventing serious complications, with the possible exception of heart attacks for metformin therapy.

Perhaps the problem is not so much with the drugs themselves, but with the mindset of the users. When people take drugs they often offload responsibility for healing to the drug and don't bother with lifestyle changes. Powerful drugs like antibiotics reinforce this mindset. When we take an antibiotic for an infection it may come with instructions to get lots of rest and drink plenty of fluids. Even if we ignore the advice, the antibiotic normally clears up the infection anyway. It doesn't work this way with today's diabetes medications. The advice to exercise and eat properly cannot be safely ignored; no matter how many pills or shots one is taking. As patients too often forget, diabetes drug therapy may complement diet and exercise, but it is no substitute for them.

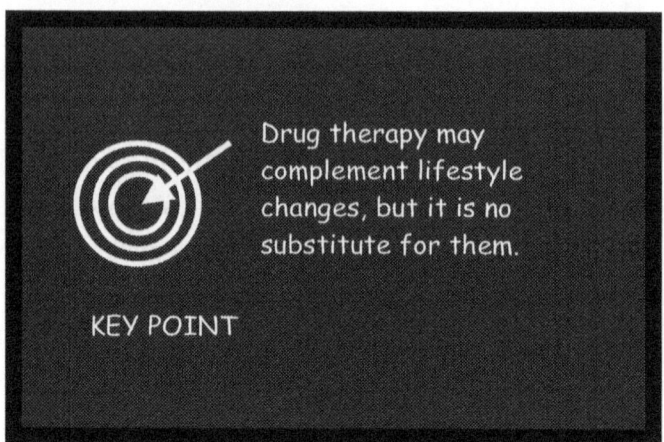

Chalkboard 9.2: Drugs are no substitute for positive lifestyle changes

Perhaps with a realistic understanding of the effectiveness of today's drugs, more patients will be motivated to make lifestyle changes and more health professionals will emphasize them. Unfortunately, the current trend is just the opposite; doctors increasingly prescribe diabetes drugs because they believe that the benefits provided outweigh the high costs and risks associated with them. Why this is, is the subject of the next chapter, Sugarcoating Healthcare.

10

Sugarcoating Healthcare

"Doctors are the third leading cause of death," read the headline of several health news articles in 2000. Whereas this emotionally charged phrase employs a good dose of *Overgeneralization*, it is important to understand where it comes from. In 2000, an article in the *Journal of the American Medical Association* reported that nearly a quarter of a million deaths per year result from causes that can be blamed on doctors: unnecessary surgery, medication errors, adverse effects of medication, infections originating in hospitals, and other medical errors.[260] When taken together as one cause of death, the annual number of "doctor caused" deaths ranks only behind heart disease and cancer.

When we sort out the various causes, we find that nearly half of these deaths were related to medication. Surprisingly, a small number (7,000) were due to medication error, while the vast majority (106,000) resulted from adverse affects of the drugs when prescribed and taken correctly. Clearly, prescription drugs are not without side effects. Every year in the U.S., prescription drug-related problems generate millions of extra visits to the doctor, emergency department visits, admissions to hospitals, admissions to long-term care facilities, and additional prescriptions resulting in an estimated cost of over *$177 billion* annually.[261,262] It has been estimated that for every dollar spent on medications another dollar is spent to treat new health problems caused by the medication.[263]

Are these problems the fault of the doctors, or the drug makers, or the FDA? The problem, as we shall see, stems from a self-reinforcing dynamic of pathological interaction among all three. Understanding this dynamic will be key to protecting ourselves from it. For that purpose, this chapter will explore how the interactions among doctors, pharmaceutical companies, and the FDA lead to sugarcoating in the healthcare setting.

Selling prescription drugs has become one of the fastest growing, most profitable businesses in the U.S. In 1993, nearly two billion prescriptions were dispensed in U.S. pharmacies. By 2001 the figure was three billion and by 2005, four billion.[264] Prescription drug sales topped half a trillion dollars in 2004, generating tens of billions in profits for pharmaceutical companies.[265,266] In terms of profit, the pharmaceutical industry dwarfs most other sectors. In 2002, the top ten pharmaceutical companies made more profit than the other 490 Fortune 500 companies combined.[267]

The key to increased profits is marketing, and the pharmaceutical companies do not skimp in this area. On average, the pharmaceutical industry spends about one third of its half trillion dollar annual revenue marketing drugs.[268] In 2000, Merck spent over $160 million—a larger marketing budget than Budweiser or Pepsi had that year—marketing Vioxx, an anti-arthritis medication.[269] Much of that money went toward marketing directly to consumers. Anyone who lives in the U.S. has surely noticed these "ask your doctor" ads all over newspapers, magazines, television, radio, and billboards. Whereas the practice is outlawed nearly everywhere else on the planet, in the U.S. more than three billion dollars a year is spent advertising drugs to consumers.[270] Many ads attempt to create the perception that newer drugs represent a major improvement over existing drugs even when they don't. Celebrex, another heavily advertised pain medication in the same class as Vioxx, was reprimanded three times in fourteen months by the FDA for overstating the drug's effectiveness. In reality, Vioxx and Celebrex do not reduce pain and inflammation more effectively than ibuprofen, and are only slightly less likely to cause pain or ulcers.[271] Clinical trial data indicating that these drugs are more likely to cause heart attacks led to the early stoppage of two trials involving Vioxx and Celebrex in 2004.

Direct to consumer advertising is a useful tool for creating new markets for drugs. Drug companies have been very successful at convincing people with mild everyday conditions that they have a clinically serious medical problem that must be treated with drugs. We've already seen how cholesterol lowering medications became the number one selling class of drugs in the U.S. thanks to *Overgeneralization* from a select group of responders to just about anyone with higher than average cholesterol. Nowadays, we have Zoloft for anyone who has had a bad day, Ritalin for misbehaving children, and Levitra, which is apparently suitable for anyone who watches sports. The recent marketing of erectile dysfunction drugs to women demonstrates where the pharmaceutical industry draws the line in using *Overgeneralization* to sell drugs.

Another way *Overgeneralization* is used to expand the market for a drug is marketing the drug for off-label uses, i.e., uses for which it is not FDA-approved. While doctors can legally prescribe drugs for off-label uses, it is not legal for a company to market them as such. Nonetheless, it is routinely done because it can expand a market several-fold for a drug that has been approved for a single niche use.

The drug Neurontin, which was approved only as an add-on therapy for epilepsy, has generated several billion dollars in revenue from more than a dozen off-label uses including diabetic neuropathy. The aggressiveness with which Neurontin was marketed for off-label uses is illustrated in the words of a senior marketing executive:

> *I want you out there every day selling Neurontin. Look this isn't just me, it's come down from Morris Plains that Neurontin is more profitable. ... We all know Neurontin's not growing adjunctive therapy, beside that is not where the money is. Pain management, now that's money. Monotherapy, that's money. We don't want to share these patients with everybody, we want them on Neurontin only. We want their whole drug budget, not a quarter, not half, the whole thing... That's where we need to be holding their hand and whispering in their ear: 'Neurontin for pain, Neurontin for monotherapy, Neurontin for everything.'* [272]

This quote and a mound of evidence of illegal marketing practices comes from a lawsuit filed by insider Dr. David Franklin, who worked as a "medical liaison" to motivate other doctors to prescribe Neurontin for off-label uses. Franklin says he was trained to exaggerate the results of scientifically weak studies, like the one about diabetic neuropathy (*Glorification*) and hide evidence that Neurontin wasn't safe or effective (*Selective Omission*).[273,274] Neurontin's makers pled guilty to paying doctors tens and even hundreds of thousands of dollars to endorse off-label uses of Neurontin to other physicians, who were often paid to attend dinners, meetings, and seminars.

Pharmaceutical companies spend the vast majority of their marketing budgets on doctors since it is the doctors' prescribing habits that will ultimately determine the sales of a drug. Each year the pharmaceutical industry spends over ten billion dollars on free samples and another six billion (roughly fifteen thousand per physician) on gifts, dinners, travel, and cash in the form of "consulting" fees (often paid to physicians to pitch or hear about a drug).[275,276,277]

<u>Ways to Influence Doctors</u>

- Travel, entertainment, & meal$
- $ponsorship
- $cholarships and educational funds
- Research grant$
- Gratuitie$
- $witching fees
- con$ulting fees

Chalkboard 10.1: Ways to influence doctors

Do these billions pay back by influencing doctors to prescribe more expensive drugs regardless of their safety and efficacy? Hundreds of studies say yes. While doctors may not think they're being influenced, the studies show that doctors who see company reps (and eighty to ninety five percent do) are more likely to add new drugs to the hospital formulary, prescribe the newer drugs, and to comply with patients' requests for medication even if they don't need it.[278,279,280] The large sums of money that drug companies spend on doctors pay back several-fold in the form of increased name-brand prescription expenditures and irrational and incautious prescribing.[281]

A common form of marketing to physicians involves regular visits from sales representatives who bring pens, pads, coffee mugs, free samples, and often lunch along with a sales pitch for some drug. This process is known as "detailing." It's no wonder the doctors often seem short on time; on average, they receive ten visits a week from drug sales reps.[282] There are approximately ninety thousand drug sales representatives currently roaming the halls of hospitals and doctors offices; that's about one for every five or six doctors.[283]

Fortunately, conscientious physicians try to look past the freebies and sales pitches of the detailers and make their prescribing decisions based on scientific evidence. That is why drug marketing firms go to great lengths to influence the doctor's primary sources of information: continuing medical education, published research, and other doctors.

Continuing medical education (CME) hours are required in most states for doctors to maintain their medical licenses. Many doctors attend educational lectures, seminars, and conferences willingly, especially when their expenses are paid by drug companies. Of the more than a billion dollars spent annually on educating physicians, most of the funding for comes from the marketing budgets of drug companies.[284]

In recent years, an increasing amount of continuing medical education programs are being developed and put on by medical education and communication companies (MECCs). MECCs compete with each other for drug company clients based on their ability to communicate the client's message and increase sales through professional education. Many blatantly advertise their services as "education and promotion."

Drug company bias in medical education is so pervasive that the Accreditation Council for Continuing Medical Education (ACCME) receives about one complaint a week from doctors and each year finds several accredited providers out of compliance with their standards.[285] When a promotional MECC is ACCME-accredited it can develop educational programs without review by an accredited body; anything it says is considered accredited medical education. As Hugh Gosling, editor of *Pharmaceutical Marketing*, put it, "Medical education used to be seen as purely non-promotional. That is no longer the case."[286] The integration of medical education and product promotion is *Edumarketing* sugarcoating. The marketing is just subtle enough to make doctors feel like they are being educated, when they are actually being swayed into prescribing newer, more expensive drugs.

In a paper published in the *Journal of the American Medical Association*, Dr. Ashley Wazana reviewed data from 538 published studies related to continuing medical education. Dr. Wazana's review found the following:

- drug company sponsored continuing medical education is biased toward the sponsor's drug
- doctors who attend sponsored continuing medical education events and accept funding for travel or lodging are more likely to prescribe the sponsor's medication
- attending presentations given by pharmaceutical representative speakers is associated with non-rational prescribing

In the words of Joe Torre, executive of Torre Lazur McCann advertising agency:

Very often doctors are more influenced by what other doctors say than what pharmaceutical companies say. So companies work through medical education companies to have doctors who support their products talk about their products in a favorable way. That's called medical education.[287]

You might also call it sugarcoating in the form of *Testimoney*. When doctors are paid to endorse drugs to other doctors, they are hardly providing an unbiased professional opinion, but are giving a sponsored sales pitch. This is not unlike the marketing technique employed by celebrities when they are secretly paid by pharmaceutical companies to endorse their products in television talk show spots.[288]

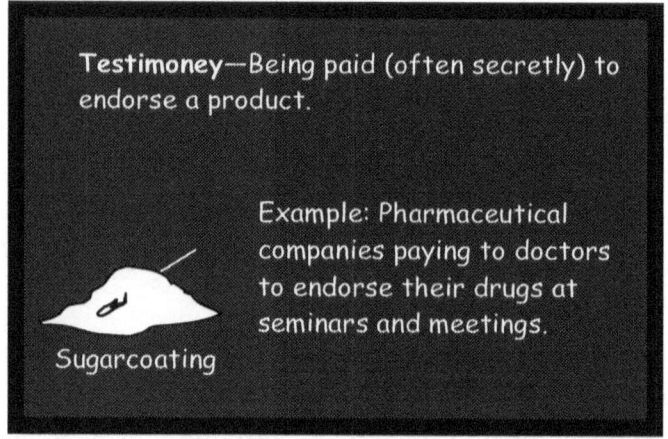

Chalkboard 10.2: Definition of Testimoney

Torre Lazur McCann, the fourth largest healthcare marketing agency in the world, is known as the 'Launch Agency' because they have successfully launched sixty-five new pharmaceutical products. They are successful because, according to Torre, "We provide services that go from the beginning of drug development all the way to the launch of your products."[289] One such service entails involvement with clinical trials, the studies that examine the effectiveness and side effects of a drug. In recent years increasing numbers of clinical trials have moved from academic health centers to contract research organizations (CROs), which are designed to run clinical trials more quickly and efficiently than university physicians. The problem with this is that, like MECCs, CROs must compete on the value they bring to their clients, the drug companies. Study outcomes that are not pleasing to the client do not tend to lead to repeat business.

It's not surprising then that company-sponsored studies are four to five times more likely to have outcomes favoring the sponsor.[290,291] Drug companies exercise control over data, control over publication, and other well-documented methods to achieve marketing objectives with clinical trials.[292,293] Often the CROs send report forms back to the sponsoring company, which performs the data analysis. Scientific papers are written by hired professional ghostwriters working under the supervision of the drug company and are handed to academic researchers to sign their names and present at conferences. The drug companies sponsor the conferences and influence which papers are presented at the conferences. Presenters and planted audience members engage in *Glorification*, *Overgeneralization*, and *Testimoney*. Doctors are influenced and drugs prescribed, providing drug companies with a handsome return on their CRO and MECC investments.

In November of 2002, the *New York Times* told the revealing story of a drug company that used a CRO to increase sales. Bextra is a drug that was rejected by the FDA for treatment of acute pain. In a quandary over how to distinguish Bextra from the crowded market of regular prescription pain relievers, its marketers came up with a strategy to generate sales from off-label uses. Having doctors and sales reps push off-label uses is punishable, as we saw with Neurontin, so the strategy for Bextra would be different: let clinical research do it. The makers of Bextra outsourced a clinical trial examining Bextra's effectiveness against acute dental pain to a CRO named Scirex. Scirex's study produced exactly the results the drug company was looking for and the results were published in the *Journal of the American Dental Association.* The strategy worked; Bextra's sales went up 60 percent in the next three months thanks in great part to the newly publicized off label uses.

According to the *New York Times* article, Scirex slanted the study's results toward the desired conclusion. To make Bextra appear more effective, they compared a small dose of the comparison drug to a full dose of Bextra (*Minification*). To make Bextra appear safe, the drug was tested on a population whose average age was twenty-three even though Bextra's target market was significantly older (*Overgeneralization*). Few side affects were observed in this healthy, young population, but when Bextra did reach its target market, reports of serious adverse effects including life-threatening risks related to skin reactions began to surface.[294]

Scirex is a wholly owned subsidiary of Omnicom, one of the world's leading drug advertising companies. Omnicom also owns Proworx, a MECC involved in the Neurontin off-label marketing scheme.[295] Ownership of CROs and MECCs by marketing companies is a recent trend in the ever-extending reach of pharmaceutical marketing. According to the *New York Times* article, the three largest drug advertising companies had already spent tens of millions of dollars to buy or invest in CROs.[296] When pharmaceutical advertising agencies can influence or completely control a research organization's board of directors the field is ripe for sugarcoating.

In a published review of fifty-six industry-sponsored studies of nonsteroidal anti-inflammatory drugs, not one found the competitor's drug more effective than sponsor's (nearly half employed *Minification* of the competitor's dosage).[297,298] Drug companies choose not to fund clinically important studies if the results might harm sales and they choose not to publish or delay publication of unfavorable results. Their data is heavily guarded, allowing them to discard subjects having negative outcomes and control the results that are presented to the FDA. *Selective Omission*, history shows, can have devastating health consequences. Over a period of 42 years, the tobacco industry spent over $220 million funding over 1,500 scientific studies, yet not one published study found a relationship between tobacco and lung cancer, heart disease, or any other illness.

The only real threat to the pharmaceutical industry is federal regulation. To address this "problem," the pharmaceutical industry spends more on political influence than any other industry in America. During the 1999-2000 election cycle, drug companies spent $262 million on lobbying, issue ads, and campaign contributions.[299] In 2004 over twelve hundred lobbyists were listed as representing pharmaceutical corporations (that's more than two for every member of congress).[300]

What has the largest lobbying operation in America accomplished? The long list has been enumerated by The Center For Public Integrity.[301] Here are just a few highlights:

- stronger patent protection laws and weakened enforcement of marketing regulations
- an effective blockade on importation of less expensive drugs from other countries
- a Medicare drug benefit prohibiting Medicare from negotiating lower drug prices[302]

The drug companies claim that reducing drug prices would stifle innovation. True, lower prices might hinder their innovativeness in marketing products to consumers, influencing doctors, and controlling clinical trials, but as for developing new drugs, most of that research is funded by U.S. taxpayers. The National Institutes of Health spends over a billion dollars a year on medical research, providing the basic research for nearly every top-selling drug.[303,304] By taking away the government's ability to bargain collectively for drugs, taxpayer money that could otherwise go to innovative research is going toward prime time advertising, physician travel expenses, detailers, lobbyists, lawyers, and consultants whose job it is to make sure things run smoothly at the FDA.

Having advocates within the FDA is another important strategic component in getting drugs to market. That is why pharmaceutical companies frequently hire ex-FDA officials as consultants to leverage their relationships with current FDA officials. Former drug company employees and board members frequently hold administrative appointments within the government. This rotation of personnel between government and industry is known around Washington as the pharmaceutical industry revolving door.

The result of pharmaceutical company influence on the FDA is that harmful drugs are quick to be approved and are slow to be withdrawn. A survey of FDA medical officers found twenty-seven instances in which a drug was approved over their objection.[305] In many instances FDA doctors were told not to present data that might adversely affect the chance of a drug being approved. In February 2005, when an FDA advisory committee, made up of thirty-two scientists, voted to keep Bextra, Celebrex, and Vioxx on the market, it was discovered that ten of the voting panelists were affiliated with the manufacturers of these drugs.[306] If these scientists with conflicts of interest had been excluded from the vote, the decision would have gone the other way.

David Graham, a senior FDA drug safety specialist, in his testimony on Vioxx said, "The FDA, as currently configured, is incapable of protecting America against another Vioxx. We are virtually defenseless. [...] What has happened with Vioxx is really a symptom of something far more dangerous to the safety of the American people."

Graham should know; he's been at the FDA for more than twenty years and has worked, often against stiff opposition from FDA officials, to get several harmful drugs withdrawn. One of those was a diabetes drug called Rezulin, which was finally withdrawn in 2000 after killing or injuring thousands of patients.[307] The story of corruption, greed, and heroism surrounding the approval and ultimate recall of Rezulin is told in our next chapter.

11

The Story of Rezulin

Most of the time, the public has no way of knowing what goes on behind closed doors between pharmaceutical companies and FDA officials. However, thanks to a series of investigative articles written by David Willman of the *Los Angeles Times*, the story of the diabetes drug Rezulin was made public knowledge and the damage caused by Rezulin was ultimately stopped. As patients and healthcare workers who deal with type 2 diabetes, it is important to know the story of Rezulin so we can protect ourselves from experiencing such a tragedy again. The story, as told in this chapter, is largely based on the information reported in Willman's series of articles.

In the late 1990's, Warner-Lambert's Rezulin had the makings of a Wall Street darling. It was the first of a new class of diabetes drugs, thiazolidinediones (TZDs), aimed at improving insulin sensitivity. Shareholders and Wall Street analysts were excited by Rezulin's "new mechanism of action" and the expanding market of type 2 diabetes patients. "[Rezulin] has the potential to virtually redefine the diabetes market and the therapeutic options open to million of patients around the world." said Lodewijk J.R. de Vink, Warner-Lambert President and Chief Operating Officer.[308]

Before Rezulin came along, Warner-Lambert was a medium

sized company sporting a solid line of consumer health products including Halls cough drops and Listerine mouthwash. Its pharmaceutical business was not faring as well, however. Revenues had fallen considerably due to competition from generics and the company was being prosecuted for concealing from the FDA deficiencies in its drug manufacturing process, a felony. In November of 1995, Warner-Lambert pleaded guilty to the charges and agreed to pay a ten million dollar fine.[309]

That same month Warner-Lambert made one of its most profitable investments ever; the company entered a formal consulting agreement with Dr. Richard C. Eastman, the top diabetes researcher at the National Institutes of Health. Warner-Lambert used Eastman as an opinion leader and to train other opinion leaders recruited by the company. Eastman was paid consulting fees to be a faculty member of the "Rezulin National Speakers Bureau," a group that urged doctors to prescribe the drug (*Testimoney*), and to serve on the education council of the "National Diabetes Education Initiative," an organization whose lecture materials recommended Rezulin (*Edumarketing*).[310] Both groups were funded by Warner-Lambert.

Eastman was an extremely valuable asset because he oversaw the Diabetes Prevention Program, a large government-funded study of the effectiveness of various treatments at preventing diabetes. Being selected to participate in the Diabetes Prevention Program would give Rezulin a great head start on the road to blockbuster stardom. Fortunately for Warner-Lambert, Eastman also oversaw the selection of drugs to be used in the study.

In June 1996 Rezulin was selected for use in the Diabetes Prevention Program and shortly thereafter became the first diabetes drug granted a six-month, fast track review by the FDA under the then brand-new US Food and Drug Modernization Act. However, getting Rezulin approved by the FDA would present a number of challenges.

In early studies, animals given doses of Rezulin had discolored, overweight hearts.[311] To satisfy FDA concerns about Rezulin's effect on human hearts, Warner-Lambert conducted the Echo study, so called for its use of echocardiograms. Only patients with a relatively normal heart function were selected to participate in the trial. After forty-eight weeks none of the patients who completed the study experienced heart failure. However, twenty-six percent of the subjects had dropped out. The FDA took a closer look and found disturbing differences in how Warner-Lambert's consultants interpreted the same echocardiogram data.[312] The problems were cleared up by FDA decisions to accept the opinion of Warner-Lambert's central reader and to exclude a data set, which had evidence of enlarged hearts, on the grounds of "poor local technique."[313]

In human clinical trials, liver injury was five times more prevalent in patients taking Rezulin than in placebo-treated patients.[314] This difference would have made Rezulin far too liver-toxic to be approved, so this information was not disclosed to the FDA. Instead, materials provided to the FDA advisory committee stated that the incidence of liver injury was "lower for [Rezulin]-treated patients compared to placebo" (*Manufacting*).[315] Warner-Lambert's vice president for diabetes research, Dr. Randall W. Whitcomb, told the committee that occurrences of liver injury among Rezulin patients were "comparable to placebo" in the clinical studies and assured them that additional liver-related data, to be furnished within days to the FDA, were "very, very similar."[316]

Even without the real data on liver injury, there was enough evidence for Dr. John Gueriguian, the FDA medical officer initially assigned to evaluate Rezulin, to recommend that Rezulin be rejected, warning of potential liver and heart risks. Unhappy with Gueriguian's report, Warner-Lambert complained to Gueriguian's boss, Dr. G. Alexander Fleming. Shortly thereafter, Fleming had Gueriguian removed from the evaluation of Rezulin and Gueriguian's medical review purged from agency files. Fleming assured Warner-Lambert's vice president for regulatory affairs Irwin G. Martin that "John is out of the picture."[317] In an internal email dated *two weeks before* Gueriguian's removal, Martin wrote, "We're over the JG hurdle."[318]

With the Echo study data revised, liver injury data withheld, and Gueriguian's review banished, Warner-Lambert had successfully leveraged FDA relationships to remove all obstacles that could prevent Rezulin from being approved at the December 11, 1996 FDA advisory committee meeting. However, there was still the issue of the "very, very similar" liver toxicity data that Warner-Lambert had promised the FDA. The data that Warner-Lambert supplied this time was far from similar; it reported a 2.2 percent rate of liver injury in Rezulin takers —almost *four times greater* than placebo.

This difference is huge for a clinical trial. Entire fields of drug therapy have been launched based on much smaller differences. Consider, for example, the pivotal Lipid Research Clinics study, which provided the celebrated "evidence" that cholesterol-lowering medication reduces risk for heart disease. In that study a nineteen percent relative reduction was exciting enough to launch the multi-billion dollar cholesterol lowering medication industry.[319] By comparison, the seventy-three percent gap between Rezulin and placebo was downplayed as "very, very, similar." By this standard, the data showing a breakthrough reduction in heart disease would be very, very, very, very, very similar. The bar charts shown in Chalkboard 12.1 illustrate how words are used to sugarcoat results.

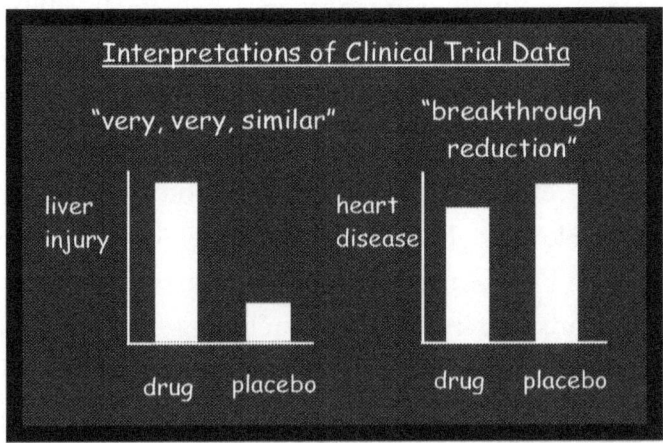

Chalkboard 12.1: Rezulin liver injury data and heart disease reduction data from LRC trial

Despite the risks Rezulin posed, the FDA advisory committee members, many of whom were on the Warner-Lambert payroll, unanimously recommended approval of the drug. When the approval was announced, Warner-Lambert's shares soared to a then all-time high on the New York Stock Exchange and a major marketing campaign began. Full-page, color magazine advertisements, including one that ran in the May 1, 1997, *New England Journal of Medicine* described Rezulin as a drug with breakthrough effectiveness and "side effects comparable to placebo." Liver toxicity was addressed as follows:

> *During all clinical studies in North America (N=2510 patients), a total of 20 Rezulin treated patients were withdrawn from treatment because of liver function test abnormalities.*[320]

This ad employed *Minification* by drawing attention to the number of patients withdrawn. A dated computer printout showed that by the time Rezulin hit the market there were seventy-eight known cases of liver injury among the 2510 clinical trial patients.[321] This would put the rate of liver injury at 3.1%, much higher than the 2.2% that was reported to the FDA or the 0.8% implied by the Rezulin ad.

As Rezulin clinical trials continued, more patients turned up with severely elevated liver enzymes. After only six months of marketing Rezulin, Warner-Lambert had received thirty-five post-marketing reports of liver injury including two cases of liver failure. Rather than pull the drug off the market, Warner-Lambert responded by lobbying the FDA to add a recommendation for short-term liver monitoring to the product label. The day before Warner-Lambert would present this proposal to the FDA, Dr. Whitcomb told the FDA that only forty-eight patients had been detected with liver injury, when in fact there were at least seventy-eight.[322] Relying on this data, the FDA accepted Warner-Lambert's recommendation to change the label, with the new language calling the incidence of liver failure "very rare."

Another key part of Warner-Lambert's strategy was getting a letter of endorsement from the director of the NIH's diabetes division, their consultant advocate Richard C. Eastman. Eastman wrote the FDA about the use of Rezulin in the Diabetes Prevention Program saying, "We continue to think that the drug is safe. ... The risk to benefit ratio in the trial continues to be one that we think is very acceptable."[323] Just days later, the British Medicines Control Agency reached the opposite conclusion stating, "the risks of [Rezulin] therapy outweigh the potential benefits" and Rezulin was promptly withdrawn from the U.K. market.[324]

In the U.S. the Rezulin label was again changed, increasing the frequency of recommended liver monitoring. The FDA issued a statement saying, "The increased monitoring of patients taking Rezulin is designed to detect those few patients in whom use of the drug can lead to serious liver damage ..."[325]

There was no scientific proof that liver monitoring would protect Rezulin patients. In fact, evidence to the contrary came when Audrey LaRue Jones, a healthy *non-diabetic* woman participating in the Rezulin arm of the Diabetes Prevention Program, died from liver failure despite undergoing strict monitoring of her liver functions. Although Warner-Lambert issued a news release saying that she died as the result of complications unrelated to Rezulin (*Ignorisolation*), NIH physicians decided the most likely cause of the liver failure was Rezulin, as did the coroner's report.

After several years of work and having spent tens of millions of dollars of public funds, the NIH decided to immediately discontinue the Rezulin arm of the Diabetes Prevention Program. With the news of this decision, the UK recall, and a steady stream of liver damage reports, some doctors began recommending increased liver monitoring beyond what the Rezulin label recommended. There was a real possibility that the FDA would mandate another labeling change requiring increased liver monitoring.

Such a mandate would have attenuated Rezulin's blockbuster sales. To deal with the matter, Warner-Lambert sent executive Irwin G. Martin to a drug industry trade group gathering to talk with FDA official Mac Lumpkin. Shortly thereafter the FDA abandoned the idea of recommending increased monitoring and continued to assure doctors that Rezulin could be used safely.

However, the news of Rezulin's toxicity had spread to consumer advocates, who began to get involved. In July 1998 consumer group Public Citizen petitioned the FDA to ban Rezulin because attempts to prevent liver damage had clearly failed. At the time of Audrey LaRue Jones' death, the FDA had received more than five hundred reports of liver toxicity due to Rezulin, twenty-one of which were fatal. Many of the deaths from liver toxicity occurred after the most recent label change, which suggested that the label changes weren't working. The FDA answered with yet another labeling change requiring increased liver monitoring.

To alleviate growing concern about the safety of Rezulin, Warner-Lambert wrote doctors a reassuring letter claiming that the label changes were working. Warner-Lambert executive Stephen J. Mock stated publicly on December 17, 1998 that, "the reported events relating to ... deaths or liver transplants since the label was changed July 28 is zero." This is another case of *Manufacting*; the number of deaths Warner-Lambert had actually reported during that time was thirty-one.[326]

The next day a participant in a Rezulin clinical trial suffered liver failure and died. As a study participant, Rosa Delia Valenzuela's liver functions were closely monitored. Her liver test results were normal when she began using Rezulin on Oct. 9, 1998 and again after the first month of treatment. By Thanksgiving, however, her liver enzymes were more than thirty times normal and she was dead before Christmas.

Warner-Lambert wrote a letter to the physicians involved in the study that Rosa had participated in for a brief ten weeks. The letter mentioned the fatality, but not how monitoring had failed to prevent it. Instead, the letter pointed to factors other than Rezulin (*Ignorisolation*). However, Rosa's death certificate stated that

Rezulin probably caused her liver failure and her liver specialist, physician, and specialists consulted by Warner-Lambert all concurred.

With doctors now becoming concerned about malpractice suits related to Rezulin, Warner-Lambert offered to provide experienced lawyers and to cover lawsuit-related expenses to keep the doctors prescribing Rezulin. The company persisted in reassuring the FDA that the number of liver-related deaths linked to Rezulin had declined dramatically from the previous year even though liver-related fatalities linked to Rezulin had actually quadrupled from the previous year.[327]

The *Los Angeles Times* investigative series of articles on Rezulin raised public awareness, and prompted an FDA reevaluation of Rezulin in January 1999. David Graham, the FDA's leading specialist in evaluating and preventing deaths caused by prescription drugs, was assigned to lead the investigation. Graham presented his findings to an FDA advisory committee meeting on March 26, 1999. He found that an estimated 430 or more Rezulin patients had suffered liver failure, that Rezulin patients incur a 1200 times greater risk of liver failure, and that more than ninety-nine percent of patients taking Rezulin for four months or longer were not undergoing the recommended liver-monitoring. These numbers made Rezulin one of the most dangerous drugs on the market. Warner-Lambert countered that preexisting medical conditions, not Rezulin, were responsible for many of the liver failures (*Ignorisolation*). The FDA committee, the same panel that had unanimously recommended Rezulin's approval, voted, eleven to one, to keep Rezulin on the market.

Just three days later, Adrian C. Seay died at the age of thirty-seven from liver failure despite undergoing monthly liver monitoring in a Rezulin clinical trial. While the death toll continued to rise, Rezulin remained on the market for all of 1999, undergoing a fourth labeling change advising increased liver monitoring.

David Graham strengthened his efforts to convince the FDA that Rezulin should be pulled from the market. On January 6, 2000, Graham shared his findings at an FDA staff meeting, convincing several physicians to conclude that Rezulin should be promptly withdrawn. Several FDA specialists banded together in support of Graham, and nicknamed themselves the "Termites." Frustrated by the FDA bureaucracy, Graham and colleagues took the battle to new levels. On March 3, Graham sent an email addressed to fourteen FDA officials exposing the senselessness of the FDA's policy toward Rezulin. Recalling how four labeling changes did not stem the rate of deaths he wrote, "At each juncture in the management of Rezulin's liver failure risk, hindsight shows that we had little or no effect and that [Warner-Lambert's] assertions that the liver failure problem was solved, were proved false."[328]

Another Termite, FDA specialist Dr. Robert I. Misbin, wrote to federal legislators about the FDA's handling of Rezulin. "In the absence of the threat of a congressional hearing," Misbin wrote on March 3, "I see little hope of turning this around until many more patients have died."[329] Misbin's correspondence included a statement from the deputy principal investigator in the Diabetes Prevention Program and consultant to Warner-Lambert, who stated that "[Warner-Lambert] deliberately omitted reports of liver toxicity and misrepresented serious adverse events experienced by [Rezulin] patients in their clinical studies."[330] The *Los Angeles Times* coverage of the story raised awareness among the lawmakers and put even more heat on the FDA. With help from the media, the efforts of the Termites finally paid off. On Tuesday,

March 21, 2000 the FDA issued a statement disclosing that Rezulin would be immediately withdrawn from the U.S. market.

Rezulin's life ended almost exactly three years after it came on the market. In that short time, the drug generated over $2.1 billion in sales for Warner-Lambert and was implicated in at least 556 documented deaths.[331] Because, in the U.S., doctors are not required to report reactions to prescription drugs no one knows exactly how many people were killed or injured by Rezulin. Given that two million people took Rezulin, one might conservatively estimate that about forty-four thousand have experienced liver injury (using the 2.2 percent figure supplied to the FDA by Warner-Lambert). To date, more than thirty-five thousand lawsuits have been filed on behalf of Rezulin users or their survivors. Pfizer, who acquired Warner Lambert in early 2000, announced that it had set aside nearly a billion dollars to settle Rezulin-related lawsuits.

The United States Attorney's office began investigating the FDA's approval of Rezulin and the money paid to government employees by Warner-Lambert. After his consulting relationship with Warner-Lambert was disclosed, Dr. Richard C. Eastman resigned from his position as diabetes researcher for the National Institutes of Health. In 2001, David Willman won a Pulitzer Prize for his investigative reporting of the Rezulin story in the *Los Angeles Times*. David Graham was named *Forbes'* Face of the Year in 2004 for his steadfast advocacy of drug safety and his willingness to blow the whistle on his bosses during the Vioxx scandal.

It took the efforts of several courageous, passionate, determined people to put an end to the damage done by Rezulin. I sometimes wonder what would have happened if the Termites hadn't fought so hard to have Rezulin removed, if David Willman was not able to obtain all the hidden documents for his investigative series of articles, or if Dr. Misbin hadn't risked losing his respected position at the FDA to write to Congressmen about Rezulin? In the absence of any of these, how long would Warner-Lambert and the FDA have let Rezulin continue to stay on the market killing and injuring diabetic patients? I am personally thankful to every one of the heroes that persisted in getting that diabetes pill off the market so I wouldn't have to take it.

12

Final Thoughts

Rezulin was still on the U.S. market when I was diagnosed with type 2 diabetes in the winter of 2000. That day I took home a bag full of free samples of diabetes drugs, including one in the same class as Rezulin. That "trick-or-treat" bag may just as easily have contained Rezulin, depending on which doctor I chose, who sponsored his last continuing medical education course, which clinical trial he was participating in, or which drug sales representative had recently taken him to lunch and dropped off free samples.

It disturbs me to know that my health and possibly my life depended on such random factors. As a layperson, knowing nothing about diabetes and blindly trusting in my healthcare team and the FDA, I would have taken whatever medicine along with whatever line of sugarcoating I was given. In fact, that's exactly what I did until I was fortunate enough to stumble upon the truth— another seemingly random event for which I am eternally grateful. That gratitude has inspired me to write this book.

I don't believe that seeing a doctor needs to be a game of Russian roulette. Prescribing treatments that *may* make you better, *may* make you worse, or *may* kill you is unacceptable. Doing so represents a step backward from the origins of modern medicine, when the practice of healing transitioned from a mystical ritual to a science-based discipline with its first precept: *do no harm*. In a relatively short time the pharmaceutical industry has reverted science-based medicine back to a mystical practice, where our faith in science is systematically exploited by a corporate marketing machine focused solely on market growth and revenue expansion. It may take several generations to repair this broken healthcare system, but an understanding of the sugarcoating can help you to use it effectively, as I have, to achieve success against diabetes.

This book has revealed the various methods of sugarcoating used to sell products to type 2 diabetics. We live in a time when relatively little is known about type 2 diabetes and most of what we hear comes from marketing messages designed to sell products. Aggressive food industry marketing convinces us to consume more unhealthy food. As we grow obese and develop chronic diseases the drug companies step in, incessantly marketing their products to patients and doctors. When patients, frustrated with high costs and lack of results, seek alternatives, the supplement industry is right there with its natural cures, all for a price of course. As we've seen, there's not a lot of substance behind the sugarcoating.

The good news is that you can avoid it by using your ability to identify sugarcoating in its various forms. You can select a good healthcare team and make positive lifestyle choices based on the best scientific information. Not all dietary advice is wrong, not all supplements are futile, and not all doctors are completely duped by the pharmaceutical industry. There are competent, knowledgeable, ethical, and up to date health professionals who are not biased by *Edumarketing* and *Testimoney*. There are unbiased sources of information. There are numerous professionals, like FDA official David Graham, who do their best to look out for your well being every day. It is critical that we find health professionals and sources of information that we can trust.

As we have learned, trust can no longer be given freely to anyone wearing a white lab coat, standing on a podium, or owning a prestigious title; it must be earned by standing up to our scrutiny. No organization is going to do this for us. When drug marketing firms own the companies that educate doctors and perform clinical trials, we must assume a greater personal responsibility for distinguishing between real information and sugarcoated marketing slogans. Indeed our survival will depend on our skepticism. Listen with a discerning mind, and determine for yourself what is right.

Remember, your greatest ally and gold standard for truth is your properly calibrated glucometer. Everything else is, at best, based on studies of how groups of *other people* responded to various treatments as compared to groups of more *other people* who did not get the same treatment. While these studies are important, remember they did not involve *you*. The fact that you have type 2 diabetes and the majority of the rest of the world doesn't should remind you that your metabolism is unique and that what works for someone else doesn't necessarily work for you. Use your meter to determine how everything—food, supplements, drugs, exercise, rest, stress, and daily activities—affects *your* body.

I hope this book will enable you to do those things more effectively by removing the biggest roadblock to your success: misinformation. I believe that seeing through the sugarcoating can have a powerful impact on your life as it has made a tremendous difference in mine. That is why I have shared what I have learned with you through this book. I hope you will share *Sugarcoating Diabetes* with others who may benefit from this information.

Appendices

Appendix A—Diabetes FAQ

A simplified, sugar-free explanation of type 2 diabetes

This appendix provides background information about type 2 diabetes that wasn't necessarily given in the main part of the book.

What are type 1 and type 2 diabetes?

The two most common types of diabetes are type 1 (about 5% of cases) and type 2 (about 95% of cases). While both types are characterized by chronically high levels of blood glucose (sugar), and the symptoms and complications are the same, the causes of type 1 and type 2 diabetes are very different.

Type 1 diabetes refers to cases characterized by complete destruction of insulin-producing cells in the pancreas; most commonly by the body's own autoimmune system. Type 1 diabetes often occurs in youth, quickly and completely destroying insulin function, and requiring patients to be insulin dependent at diagnosis.

Type 2 diabetes, which occurs most often in adults, is a metabolic disorder in which insulin function degrades gradually, so that patients typically do not require insulin at diagnosis.

For many type 2 patients, having high blood sugar is just a condition like having high cholesterol, high blood pressure, or too much body fat. Type 2 diabetes itself does not cause pain or suffering; it is the complications, which result from several years of uncontrolled blood glucose, that do. Type 2 diabetes typically goes unnoticed until a person reaches a dangerously high blood glucose level or complications start to become evident.

Why is it called type 2 diabetes?

The technical name is *Type 2 diabetes mellitus* (*T2DM*). The term *diabetes* is Greek, meaning literally "to pass through." It is generally agreed that the term came about from the observation that people with diabetes pee a lot. Later, when it was discovered that the pee contained a great deal of sugar the term *mellitus* (sweet) was appended. Thus the scientific name *diabetes mellitus* refers to the condition of peeing frequently with great sweetness.

The prefix *type 2* is a recent innovation indicating that, as much as we'd like to think we know what this disease is all about, we're still fairly clueless. If we had a clue, we might drop the sweet pee moniker and call it something like *amylinoma* or *beta cell anemia* or even something more fun like *Langerhanzers disease*. Instead the name *type 2 diabetes* just indicates some vague distinction from the equally non-descriptive type 1 diabetes.

Type 1 and type 2 used to be distinguished by the slightly more descriptive terms *juvenile* and *adult onset*. Those names, however, didn't tell us anything about the diseases themselves, just how old the patients tended to be at diagnosis. Since it turned out that a large number of adults have juvenile diabetes and many juveniles get the adult onset type, the names were changed in 1979 to *Insulin Dependent Diabetes Mellitus* (*IDDM*) and *Non-Insulin Dependent Diabetes Mellitus* (*NIDDM*). These names, however, didn't tell us anything about the diseases either, just what treatments tended to be used. The new names were confusing, especially when a patient's treatment was changed though their disease obviously didn't. Such conundrums led to the invention of terms like *Insulin Dependent Non-Insulin Dependent Diabetes Mellitus* (*IDNIDDM*). Try pronouncing that. In 1999 the scientific community realized that these names were awful and retreated to the *type 1* and *type 2* we use today.

How well are we controlling type 2 diabetes?

Not very well. Type 2 diabetes has been declared an epidemic in the United States and is on the rise in all age groups. From 1990 to 1998 the prevalence of diagnosed diabetes in U.S. adults rose from 4.9% to 6.5%, an increase of 33%.[332] In the next year, 1999, it shot up to 6.9%, rising almost as much as Ebay stock did that year.[333] Despite the fact that we have more knowledge, more drugs, and better self-monitoring tools than ever, the problem appears to be getting worse, not better.

What are the symptoms of type 2 diabetes?

Symptoms of high blood glucose are extreme thirst, frequent urination, genital itching (yeast infection), and sudden weight loss. Symptoms that complications are setting in include blurry vision and numbness or tingling in the legs.

What is pre-diabetes?

Having pre-diabetes means one has higher than normal blood sugar, but not enough to meet the cutoff for type 2 diabetes. Pre-diabetes and type 2 diabetes lie on a continuum of degrees of severity, like high cholesterol, high blood pressure, and high body fat. Much like these conditions, type 2 diabetes is clinically defined by an arbitrary cutoff point, which many patients regularly cross in both directions. The term "pre-diabetes" pessimistically suggests that the condition will, in time, turn into to diabetes. This is like saying an overweight person has "pre-obesity." As with gaining and losing weight, the lifestyle choices one makes can make one more or less diabetic.

There are two better-named conditions that fall under the umbrella of pre-diabetes: impaired fasting glycemia (IFG) and impaired glucose tolerance (IGT). IFG describes a condition when blood glucose in between meals is higher than normal. It is indicated when one's fasting blood glucose is above 100, but less than 126—the cutoff for type 2 diabetes. IGT describes the condition when one's glucose after meals is above normal. IGT is indicated when glucose measured two hours after a high-carbohydrate meal is above 140 but less than 200—the cutoff point for type 2 diabetes.

What is LADA?

In 2000, over one million new adults joined the type 2 diabetes club[334]. However, many of them didn't belong. They may have felt a little strange at the support group meetings because they weren't overweight and tended to be younger than the rest of the crowd. These people have *latent autoimmune diabetes of the adult (LADA)*, also known as *adult onset type 1*, or *type 1.5*. LADA patients are frequently misdiagnosed as type 2s. They often have the genes and the antibodies characteristic of type 1s but not always. Many completely lose their beta cells and require insulin, but some don't. According to the UKPDS, one-fourth of all type 2 subjects between the age of twenty-five and forty-five are LADA.

What is glucose?

Glucose is a type of sugar that is used throughout the body for energy. Normally about one teaspoon (five grams) of glucose circulates in the blood at all times to provide energy to the billions of glucose using cells. These cells consume glucose at the rate of about five teaspoons per hour. Thus the body is constantly working to keep enough glucose circulating in the blood. This is important because too little glucose can cause you to pass out, go into a coma, and die. Too much can, over time, catalyze the process that leads to complications.

Where does glucose come from?

Glucose is manufactured, stored, and released by the liver.

The liver gets its raw materials primarily from diet but can, if necessary, produce glucose from the body's fat stores and muscle tissue. Since we are not constantly eating, we typically eat enough food in a meal to supply the body with glucose for several hours afterward. After a meal, excess glucose is stored in the liver and muscle tissue and also converted into fat and stored in fat cells. These stores are used in between meals for energy and to keep circulating blood glucose levels from dropping too low.

In the average-sized person nearly a pound (four hundred grams) of glucose is stored in the muscles. The liver stores about fifteen teaspoons (seventy-five grams). When fasting, the liver releases about a teaspoon and a half (eight grams) of glucose per hour into the bloodstream. Most of that comes from its internal stores, but some from the recycling of proteins from broken down muscle tissue.

The glucose processing functions of the liver are affected by two important hormones secreted by the pancreas: insulin and glucagon. Insulin tells the liver to store glucose and glucagon tells the liver to break down its stores and release glucose into the blood. Both hormones are always present in some amount but work together to control blood glucose levels. After a meal, glucose is abundant and insulin levels are raised to keep blood glucose levels from getting too high. Between meals glucagon liberates stored glucose to keep blood glucose levels from going too low.

What is high blood sugar/glucose?

When glucagon and insulin are out of balance, so is blood sugar. If the body's insulin function is impaired, as it is in type 2 diabetes, circulating glucose is not stored and remains in the bloodstream. Too much glucagon relative to insulin can also cause the liver to release too much glucose into the bloodstream. Overproduction of glucose by the liver is common in type 2 diabetes. High blood glucose can occur when cells in the liver and muscle tissue are "resistant" to insulin; i.e., when they require more insulin than normal to do their job.

What you eat directly influences your blood glucose. Dietary carbohydrates, like sugar, flour, and starch have a much greater elevating effect on blood sugar than dietary protein and fat. Dietary protein, fat, and fiber can slow down the rate at which carbohydrates raise blood sugar.

What should my blood glucose be?

Everyone's body is different, but normal ranges have been established for two types of blood glucose measurements: fasting and post-prandial. Fasting blood glucose is a measurement taken when one has not eaten recently, for example, when waking up in the morning. Fasting blood glucose should normally be in the range of 80-100 mg/dl. Post-prandial glucose is a measurement taken two hours after a meal and is normally in the range of 100-140 mg/dl.

Average blood sugar is often estimated by the HbA1c test. The normal range for HbA1c is 4.6 to 6.4 percent.

What are HbA1c and Fructosamine?

HbA1c is just the scientific name for a type of hemoglobin, or blood protein, that has been chemically bound to glucose. This binding of glucose is called glycation and the term "glycated hemoglobin" simply refers to hemoglobin with glucose attached to it. HbA1c is a more specific term, referring to a specific type of hemoglobin molecule with glucose attached at a particular terminal on the molecule.

When you measure the percentage of HbA1c in your blood,

you know how much glycation has occurred over the last four weeks or so, which gives you an idea of how much sugar has been around in your blood during that time. Many people believe the HbA1c test measures average blood sugar over three months because hemoglobin cells die and are recycled about every ninety days. However, because there is a reverse reaction the test is heavily weighted to recent activity. HbA1c is believed to be a good estimator of fasting blood glucose but has no relationship to post-prandial glucose.[335]

HbA1c also appears to be a good indicator of the extent of damage that leads to complications. Clinical studies have shown that people with higher HbA1c scores tend to have a higher rate of complications. Keeping HbA1c below 7.0 percent is recommended to reduce the risk of complications.

Hemoglobin is just one of many proteins that can be glycated. The fructosamine test measures the glycation of plasma proteins (albumin and immunoglobulins), to indicate average blood sugar over a three-week period.

What are the complications of diabetes?

High blood glucose is believed to cause damage to many tissues of the body. Damage to small blood vessels, like those found in nerve cells, results in a variety of so-called *microvascular* complications.

One of the most common microvascular complications is neuropathy, in which nerves in the hands and feet are damaged causing loss of touch sensitivity, and allowing ulcers and other infections like gangrene to take over toes and feet. When these infections get out of control, toes, feet, and legs have to be amputated. In the United States diabetes is the leading cause of lower extremity amputations not related to injury.

Damage to the autonomic nervous system can cause erectile dysfunction in men. Diabetes is the single most common cause of erectile dysfunction in the United States.

Diabetic retinopathy is a complication in which damage to the tiny vessels in the eye's retina leads to progressively worsening vision. In advanced stages new, abnormal blood vessels, which are formed on the retina in an attempt to restore normal blood flow, may rupture and bleed causing detachment of the retina and permanent vision loss. Retinal photocoagulation, a laser procedure used to seal the retina and stop vessels from growing and leaking, can prevent or delay blindness. A form of retinopathy more common in type 2 diabetes, called macular edema, involves a swelling of the macula, the part of the eye responsible for sharp, detailed vision, resulting in distorted vision. Diabetes is the leading cause of new blindness in adults in the United States.

High blood glucose in combination with other factors such as high blood pressure can lead to diabetic nephropathy. Diabetic nephropathy is a condition in which filters in the kidneys, called glomeruli, gradually fail, resulting in impaired kidney functioning. Nephropathy may eventually lead to excessive loss of protein in the urine (microalbuminuria) and ultimately kidney failure requiring dialysis. Diabetes is the leading cause of end stage renal disease (ESRD) accounting for more than half of new patients entering ESRD programs in the United States.

People with diabetes are at increased risk for *macrovascular* (large blood vessel) complications, such as atherosclerosis in the heart, stroke in the brain, and peripheral vascular disease in the extremities. Whether or not high blood sugar causes these diseases, or is merely correlated is still an open question.

What causes complications?

In diabetes, circulating blood contains elevated levels of glucose. Whereas most cells still manage to keep their internal glucose at normal levels, other cells—particularly endothelial cells that line arteries and the capillaries of the retina and kidney—are unable to regulate glucose and develop high internal levels. This in turn activates pathways of cellular damage that lead to complications. There are four known pathways to complications: the polyol pathway, the hexosamine pathway, advanced glycation end product (AGE) formation, and activation of protein kinase C. There is now good evidence that all four pathways are activated by the same event: the overproduction of superoxide in the mitochondria, which can be induced by high levels of glucose.[336,337,338]

What is insulin?

Insulin is a hormone, meaning that it is a substance manufactured and used by the body for long-distance communication between cells. Insulin is secreted by a tiny part of the pancreas called the *Islets of Langerhans*. The islets were named after the nineteen year-old medical student, Paul Langerhans, who discovered the islets but had no idea what they did. Later it was discovered that beta cells within the islets were responsible for manufacturing and secreting insulin. Insulin has numerous effects on the body, its primary ones being to tell the liver to store glucose and to tell the body's other cells to store glucose and fat.

Insulin takes the spotlight after a meal. High levels of nutrients in the blood, particularly glucose, stimulate beta cells within the islets to manufacture insulin and secrete it. The insulin goes directly to the liver, through a vein called the portal vein. The liver uses up about half of the insulin and the other half is released into general circulation. Through the circulation of blood, insulin can reach all of its target cells. Insulin signals a target cell by binding to receptors called, oddly enough, insulin receptors on the cell's surface. Each insulin-sensitive cell contains approximately a quarter of a million insulin receptors. This binding causes a cascade of activity within the cell that summons glucose transporters to the cell's membrane, resulting in the uptake of glucose and fat from the blood.

How is insulin function impaired in type 2 diabetes?

The details are not known exactly. There can be problems on the supply side, called impaired beta cell function, and on the demand side, called insulin resistance.

Impaired beta cell function means that the beta cells don't produce enough insulin to keep glucose levels in the normal range. By the time a person is diagnosed with type 2 diabetes their beta cell function is, on average, reduced by half.[339] As a result, most type 2 diabetics have an impaired ability to secrete the level of insulin necessary to regulate glucose within thirty minutes after a meal.[340,341] This leads to higher glucose levels between meals and even more work for the understaffed team of beta cells.

Insulin resistance means that the body's cells don't use insulin as efficiently as a normal person's cells would. While insulin resistance may play an important role in type 2 diabetes, it is neither necessary nor sufficient to cause it. Not all type 2 diabetics are insulin resistant and most insulin resistant people are not diabetic. Nonetheless, you may have heard a phrase like "type 2 diabetics make enough insulin, but their body is resistant to it." While this definition nicely contrasts type 2 to type 1, it suffers from the drawback of being wrong. One in three adult Americans is clinically insulin resistant and most of them produce enough insulin to keep their blood sugar under control.[342] The insulin resistant folks who make enough insulin are not diabetic, only the ones who *don't make enough* are. Thus all diabetics, by definition, do not make enough insulin.

Much of the confusion about this arose in the 1960's when the first studies with radio immunoassays (the tools used to measure insulin) produced the startling result that some type 2 diabetics have higher levels of insulin than normal weight-matched patients. However, as is often the case with science, we came to realize that we were led astray by what we didn't know. The radio immunoassays of the 1960s reacted to both proinsulin, a precursor molecule that has little effect on blood glucose, as well as insulin, leading us to overestimate the amount of useful insulin that type 2 diabetics have.[343,344] Later, when better equipment was developed, it was discovered that type 2 diabetics secrete an abnormally high fraction of proinsulin, which explains the higher readings seen with older technology, and less useful insulin.[345,346,347,348]

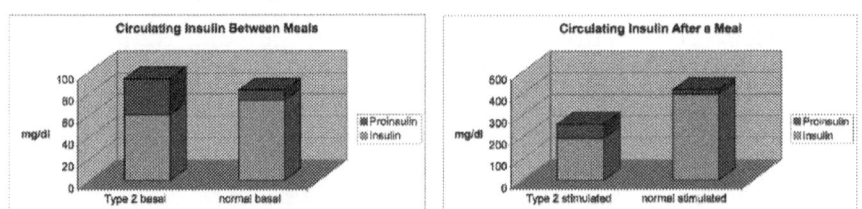

Figure A.1: Type 2 diabetics have less usable insulin than age and weight matched non-diabetics. Data from Roder et al.[349]

Figure A.1 shows clearly that type 2 diabetics have less useful insulin in circulation than non-diabetics of similar age and weight both between and after meals. The investigators in this study noted that the more diminished the capacity of the beta cells, the more proinsulin is secreted. It thus appears that the harder a beta cell has to work, the less useful insulin it produces.

Why do some insulin-resistant people become diabetic while others don't?

The common pattern of progression to type 2 diabetes occurs over a long period of time in which insulin resistance gradually increases like body weight and the beta cells compensate by producing more insulin. Eventually something causes the beta cells to start churning out less insulin and creates the diabetic state. No one knows exactly what causes this and why it only happens in some people. Scientists speculate that the beta cells may become one or more of the following:

1. *insensitive*—exposure to high levels of glucose causes beta cells to become desensitized to the glucose stimulus

2. *exhausted*—over-stimulation from glucose and/or drugs depletes the beta cells of insulin so they cannot respond to glucose even if they are fully sensitized to it

3. *dead*—reduction in number of beta cells also plays a role in impaired insulin response. Type 2 diabetics have been observed having up to sixty-three percent reduction in number of beta cells.[350]

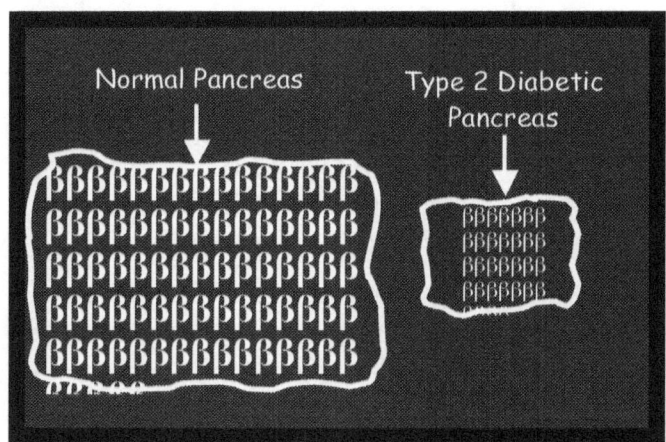

Chalkboard A.1: the diabetic pancreas has less sensitive, more exhausted, and fewer beta cells than the normal pancreas

Why do beta cells burn out?

No one knows for sure, but a leading theory is that the problem lies in the mitochondria, a key link in the chain of beta cell events that produces insulin in response to glucose.[351] An important piece of evidence for this theory came when researchers demonstrated how the mitochondrial defect leads to reduced sensitivity of the beta cell.[352] High levels of glucose overwhelm the mitochondrial electron transport system impairing insulin release.

Why do type 2 diabetics lose most of their beta cells?

Beta cells are continuously being destroyed and regenerated in the pancreas and what disturbs this delicate balance is still an open research topic. A strong body of evidence implicates high levels of glucose (glucotoxicity), free fatty acids (lipotoxicity)' and amylin (amyloidogenic toxicity) as destructive forces.[353,354,355] We also know that elevated levels of glucose, free fatty acids, and amylin are also byproducts of defective beta cell function, so the cause-effect relationships may be cyclic. Diabetes appears to be a self-inducing disease, which progresses if not controlled. Chalkboard A.2 illustrates this vicious cycle.

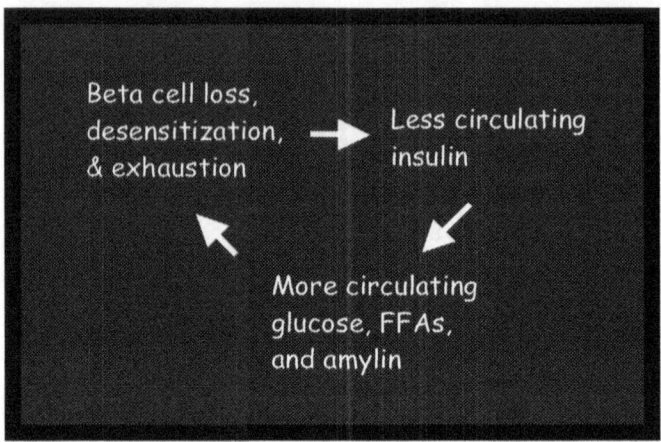

Chalkboard A.2: The vicious cycle of diabetes

How can this cycle be reversed?

The problem is normally addressed by action on multiple fronts.

Increase insulin—injecting insulin or using drugs that stimulate insulin production can normalize blood sugars and free fatty acids.

Reduce demand for insulin—a diet consisting of fewer carbohydrates and calories will reduce the demand for insulin and lower blood glucose and free fatty acids.[356,357,358,359,360,361,362]

Improve insulin sensitivity—like your weight, insulin resistance can be reduced. Exercise has a positive effect on insulin resistance and each session has an immediate effect that lasts up to 16 hours.[363,364,365] Some drugs may also improve insulin sensitivity.

When glucose levels are brought closer to normal, the liver becomes more sensitive to glucose and insulin,[366] beta cell sensitivity starts improving within as short as 20 hours,[367] insulin response improves,[368,369,370] and beta cell loss due to glucotoxicity subsides.[371] Positive changes stimulate more positive changes, bringing the whole system back into balance.

What are free fatty acids?

Fatty acids are the building blocks of fat molecules, which are called triglycerides. When triglycerides are burned for fuel, they are broken down into fatty acids, which provide energy to cells. When fatty acids are not attached to a triglyceride, they are called free fatty acids. Most cells can use either glucose or free fatty acids for energy, with the notable exception being brain cells, which cannot use free fatty acids directly.

What is amylin?

Amylin is a hormone that is secreted with insulin and, it is believed, must somehow work with insulin to stimulate glucose metabolism. Amyloid deposits are found in the islet cells of most diabetics. In 1987, the precursor to these deposits was discovered, and it was named amylin.

What is statistically significant?

When scientists observe a noticeable difference in outcomes—for example, when patients taking a drug have fewer heart attacks than those taking a placebo—they want to know whether their observation was due to the drug or just chance. The situation is analogous to a casino pit boss observing a winning gambler and wanting to know whether the player has some edge or is just lucky. If a player is winning after a few minutes of play, the pit boss will think nothing of it, assuming that the player is just lucky. However, if the player consistently stays ahead of the house after several hours of play, then the pit boss may begin to think that the player possesses a real edge. The longer the player stays ahead of the house, the less likely it appears his winning is due to chance and the more suspicious the pit boss becomes.

A study is considered statistically significant when the probability of it being produced by chance is small, usually less than .005 or a one-in-two hundred chance. The more samples one has, the less likely the observation is due to chance and the more likely it is due to a real difference.

For example, let's say you want to determine if blowing on a pair of dice before you roll it gives you a greater chance of getting a seven. You might roll the dice ten times without blowing and get one seven. Then you roll them ten times with blowing and get two sevens—a 100% improvement! But, the probability of getting this result purely by chance is quite high (the probability of rolling two or more sevens in ten rolls is better than 50/50), so your results are not statistically significant. There's a decent chance that the next time you repeat this experiment you might observe two sevens without blowing and only one seven with. However, if you did the same experiment rolling the dice 10,000 times and you got twice as many sevens blowing than not blowing, then the probability of this happening due to chance is very small. You have a statistically significant result and should head to Las Vegas immediately.

Appendix B—Supplements for Diabetes

This appendix summarizes the evidence (or lack thereof) for several supplements marketed to diabetics. The list is not comprehensive as the number of supplements purported to treat diabetes is large and growing. However, it does include most supplements for which a good body of evidence involving the treatment of diabetes exists.

Vitamins and Minerals are essential nutrients for proper functioning of the human body. The US Dietary Reference Intakes (DRIs) provide guidelines in minimal dosage. The *Recommended Dietary Allowance (RDA)* and *Adequate Intake (AI)* tell us the level of nutrient intake needed to prevent diseases in nearly all healthy people. Like healthy people, diabetics need to get *at least* the RDA or AI of each vitamin and mineral for their particular sex and age group. Levels above the RDA or AI may provide added benefits to people with diabetes.[372,373,374,375,376,377,378,379,380,381]

One class of nutrients that has been widely examined in the treatment of diabetes is the **antioxidant** group, which includes vitamin E, vitamin C, beta carotene, alpha lipoic acid, selenium, and zinc. Oxidation is a natural and vital process in the body that can be harmful when not kept in balance. In fact, excessive oxidation appears to play a key role in the development of diabetic complications.[382,383,384,385,386] Accordingly, there has been interest in prescribing antioxidants to people with diabetes.[387,388,389] However, not all antioxidants work the same way, on the same molecules, or in the same places. Different antioxidants can work together in a chain that requires a delicate balance to work optimally; an imbalance may cause an antioxidant to become pro-oxidant. To say the least, the interactions between the body's varied oxidative pathways and the different types of antioxidants are complex and not yet fully understood.

Results from antioxidant studies have been mixed. Some studies have shown health benefits in those who consume more vitamin C and vitamin E, either by taking supplements or through diet,[390,391,392] but others don't.[393,394,395] The results may be mixed because people who get their vitamins from fruits and vegetables get additional health benefits from the hundreds of other phytochemicals these foods contain. Remember, there is no substitute for healthy eating.

Carrots, green leafy vegetables, cantaloupe, peppers and sweet potatoes are all good sources of Vitamin A. Foods high in vitamin C include green and red peppers, strawberries, citrus fruits, and broccoli. Good natural sources of vitamin E are wheat germ oil, leafy greens, almonds, and sunflower seeds.

Vitamin E supplementation by itself has been investigated with great interest. While some studies have demonstrated no significant improvement,[396,397] others have shown vitamin E supplements to reduce oxidative stress,[398] lower glucose levels,[399] improve insulin action,[400] reduce protein glycation,[401] and prevent complications.[402,403]

All of these improvements appear to be related, and there is a theory that explains how. The theory is that high blood sugars increase the production of a powerful oxidant, so powerful in fact that it wears a big red "S" on its oxidizing chest and is known as Superoxide. Over production of this superoxide causes, through a series of events we won't describe here, a back-up in the process of glucose metabolism within the cell and an increase in activity of the known pathways to diabetic complications. One of the pathways to complications involves the glycation (attachment of glucose) of proteins. These glycated proteins bind with other proteins producing even more reactive and damaging products, called advanced glycation end products, that damage vital body parts such as the retina, nerves, kidneys and even the beta cells in your pancreas.

A familiar example of this process is the glycation of a specific type of hemoglobin, called HbA1c. The HbA1c test, which measures the percentage of glycated hemoglobin, is often thought of as an estimator of average blood sugar over several weeks, but it has an even more important purpose. It provides insight into the rate at which protein damage is occurring and is thus an excellent predictor of complications. Large-scale clinical trials have shown that patients with higher HbA1c scores are more likely to experience complications.[404,405]

You may have been warned that antioxidants, by preventing glycation, will "artificially" lower HbA1c scores, making you think that your blood sugar is lower than it really is when measured on a daily basis. Such warnings represent backwards thinking; preventing complications, not high blood sugar, is the primary goal. High blood sugar is only important because it is a part of the sequence of events leading to complications. However, there are other therapeutic opportunities besides lowering glucose that target various points along the pathways from high blood sugar to complications. As our understanding of the mechanisms that cause complications improves we will begin to see more of these types of therapies emerge.

Thiamine or **vitamin B-1** supplements boost the activity of an enzyme that unclogs the backup caused by superoxide. Scientists found that administration of **Benfotiamine,** a fat-soluble form of thiamine, blocked pathways leading to diabetic complications and prevented eye and kidney damage in diabetic rats.[406,407] The supplement has been used in Germany as an over-the-counter treatment for neuropathy (nerve damage common in uncontrolled diabetics) since 1992. (Rumor has it that many Germans use it to prevent hangovers too.)

Another supplement used in Germany to treat neuropathy that is available in the U.S. is **alpha lipoic acid**. Alpha lipoic acid is a powerful antioxidant that works like kryptonite, countering the effects of superoxide as well as other oxidant molecules, the so-called band of free radicals. There is a good amount of evidence that 600 mg per day of alpha lipoic acid can improve neuropathy[408,409,410,411] and insulin sensitivity in patients with type-2 diabetes.[412,413,414]

Alpha lipoic acid is found in beef, spinach, broccoli, rice bran, and other food sources but in very small quantities. For example, a 3 oz. serving of beef kidney, the richest source of alpha lipoic acid on the planet, contains just 32 micrograms. A typical supplement pill contains five to ten thousand times that much.

Deficiencies of certain minerals, such as potassium, magnesium, zinc, and chromium, may aggravate the diabetic condition. **Magnesium** is an essential mineral that is involved in hundreds of processes in the body, including energy metabolism. Low levels of magnesium have been observed in type 1 and type 2 diabetics, especially those with poor glucose control and complications. It is not clear whether magnesium loss contributes to or is the result of diabetic complications. Magnesium deficiency has been corrected with supplementation; however, no improvement in glucose control was observed.[415] In one trial supplementation with 1000 mg of magnesium lowered fructosamine levels, but 500 mg did not.[416]

Dietary sources of magnesium include whole grains, leafy green vegetables, legumes, nuts, and fish.

Chromium is perhaps the most over-hyped and consequently the most controversial supplement marketed to diabetics. Chromium is a mineral that is generally believed to be nutritionally essential, though no one knows exactly what it does. It is thought to play a role in carbohydrate metabolism by enhancing or increasing the action of insulin. This sounds potentially useful to diabetics and considerable attention has been given to studying it and even more attention to marketing it.

In large-scale studies conducted in China and Finland, supplementation with chromium at levels eight to forty times the adequate intake value decreased glucose levels and HbA1c in type 2 diabetics.[417,418] However, other studies performed on type 2 diabetics in Tunisia, the US and Israel have shown no effect on glucose levels or HbA1c.[419,420,421,422] One explanation for the mixed results is that supplementation only has a positive effect on those whose diets are deficient in chromium, and it would appear that westerners are not. However, a study from 1985 suggests that most Americans consume less than the adequate intake value and, more recently, another study found that American men with diabetes and heart disease had less toenail chromium than healthy control subjects.[423,424] These studies suggest that there might be a chromium deficiency problem in some diabetics. Whether or not chromium supplementation will help remains the subject of heated debate—one that you can settle for yourself with a bottle of chromium supplements and your meter.

Good food sources of chromium include: brewer's yeast,

peanut butter, seafood, brown rice, cheese, meat, potatoes (with skin), mushrooms, broccoli, and wheat germ.

Vanadium is another trace mineral whose physiological role is not fully known. A number of small studies have examined the effects of vanadium on type 2 diabetics, with most, but not all, showing reduction in fasting glucose, HbA1c, and cholesterol and improvement in insulin sensitivity.[425,426,427,428,429,430] Side effects such as diarrhea, nausea, and flatulence were reported in a number of patients in these studies.

The amounts used in these studies, 100 mg - 150 mg, are about one thousand times the normal daily intake and body stores. The amount of vanadium required to have a positive effect may also be toxic and increase oxidative damage. Some experts do not recommend taking vanadium supplements until more is known about how this mineral affects the human body.

Fats and vegetable oils (sunflower, safflower, corn, and olive oils) are the richest sources of vanadium. It is also found in a variety of natural foods including oysters, shellfish, buckwheat, parsley, oats, rice, green beans, carrots, cabbage, mushrooms, pepper, dill, radishes, and eggs.

L-carnitine, a derivative of the amino acid lysine, plays an important role in the production of energy from fatty acids and is believed to increase insulin sensitivity. In fact, insulin sensitivity was improved over placebo in three small clinical trials where L-carnitine was given intravenously.[431,432,433] No such data exists for oral supplements however. Only 5%-15% of L-carnitine is absorbed from oral supplements, so you have to eat a large amount (5 grams) every day to make a difference.[434,435] Beef, pork, and milk are the richest dietary sources of L-carnitine. There is no vegetarian source but the body can manufacture L-carnitine if it has sufficient quantities of lysine, methionine (another amino acid), iron, vitamin C, vitamin B6, and niacin (B3).

A number of plants from India are used to treat diabetes in Ayurveda, a traditional healing system in India. *Coccinia indica* is believed to mimic the function of insulin and, in a few trials carried out in India, was been shown to have glucose lowering effects comparable to those of conventional drugs.[436,437,438] *Allium sativum* (garlic) and *Allium cepa* (onion) have not been widely studied and results have been mixed.[439] *Trigonella foenum graecum* (fenugreek) has been shown to reduce post-prandial glucose levels (perhaps due to its fiber content) in some small studies in India.[440,441,442] Ocimum sanctum (holy basil) has been shown to lower glucose in type 2 diabetics in India.[443] *Gymnema sylvestre* was shown to lower fasting blood glucose and HbA1c in type 2 patients in India.[444] *Mamordica charantia* (bitter melon) was found to improve glucose tolerance among type 2 diabetics in India in 1986.[445]

The eastern hemisphere doesn't have a monopoly on herbal remedies, however. From Mexico we have the prickly pear cactus, *Opuntia streptacantha* (nopal), which was shown to decrease fasting glucose and insulin levels in a small number of type 2 diabetics.[446] *American Ginseng* has been widely studied and has been shown to lower glucose and HbA1c in type 2 diabetics.[447,448] However, the amount of active ginseng in supplement pills claiming to have the same amount may vary by as much as a factor of 10; some brands were found to contain none at all.[449] In general, since supplements are not regulated and the FDA can closely examine only a tiny percentage of them, you will never know what's really in the bottle.

For all supplements there seems to be a consistently ambiguous pattern: while there is always just enough evidence for a supplement manufacturer to make health claims about a product, there is never enough evidence for any of these products to be considered proven effective. If supplements are to provide any benefit at all, it will be to individuals that have a deficiency.

Appendix C—The Facts About Diabetes Drugs

This appendix provides a sugar-free look at the evidence regarding the safety and efficacy of diabetes drugs. It describes diabetes drugs on the market today, and those coming down the pipeline. Rather than provide over-simplified explanations like "helps your body's cells use insulin better" it will explain what we really know and don't know about their mechanisms of action, whether they work, for *how long*, and how safe they are. We begin with the first and best diabetes drug ever discovered.

Insulin

Insulin is considered a drug because it is produced by pharmaceutical companies, sold at drug stores, and taken on a scheduled basis. However, unlike most (and before 2005 all) of the other drugs currently on the market, insulin is a naturally occurring hormone that has been around longer than man or monkeys. In fact, insulin from pigs and cows has been used to treat diabetes in humans. Although these insulins do the trick, they are not identical to human insulin and cause some people to suffer adverse reactions. Nowadays it is possible to make insulin that is chemically identical to that which a normal human pancreas produces. Thanks to advances in recombinant DNA technology, it is now possible to splice a human gene into E. coli and have the bacteria colony produce gallons of the hormone precursor, proinsulin. Using enzymes, the proinsulin is cleaved into human insulin, which is then bottled and sold for big bucks.

Insulin from needles, however, is a crude substitute for a real functioning pancreas. Injections don't provide the steady, feedback-based dosage of beta cells, which are continuously putting out insulin—large amounts in response to glucose levels after meals and a steady stream in between meals to prevent hyperglycemia. Fast-acting and slow-acting injected insulins attempt to mimic this behavior, but the fast-acting ones (e.g. Lispro) don't act fast enough (they are absorbed too slowly) and the slow-acting ones (e.g. NPH and Lente) provide too much insulin early on and not enough to get you through the night. Chalkboard C.1 illustrates the difference between injections and a real pancreas.

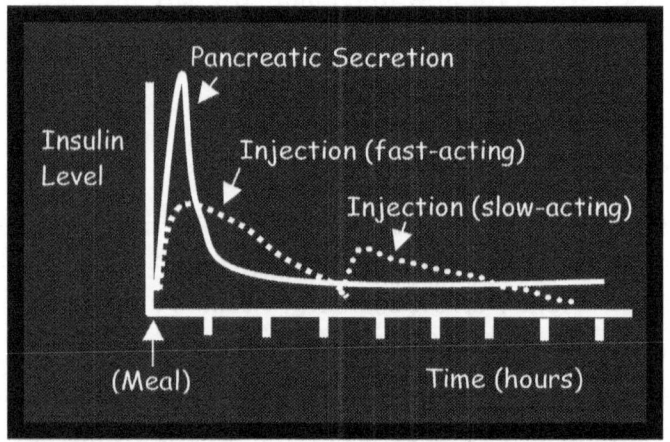

Chalkboard C.1: insulin response of pancreas (solid line) vs. injections (dashed line)

To address this problem, scientists have developed insulin analogs, which are like human insulin, only better. With a few tweaks in their chemical structure, the analogs still work like insulin but the difference can make their absorption faster than fast-acting insulin or slower than slow-acting insulin.

Fast-acting analogs, such as insulin lispro (a.k.a. Humalog) or insulin aspart (a.k.a. NovoRapid) act quickly enough that they can be injected with meals instead of before. Their action peaks at 2 hours, which is good for preventing hypoglycemia without the need for snacks, but a slow-acting insulin must be used to prevent blood sugar rise in between meals. Insulin glargine, a.k.a. Lantus, is an analog that does not peak early like NPH or Lente, but provides a steady dose for 24 hours.

While these analogs improve the situation somewhat, tight blood glucose control is still elusive because identical doses of insulin can vary in effect from day to day. Insulin absorption can vary depending on the site of injection (absorption is fastest in the abdomen, followed by the arm, then the leg), temperature, and local blood flow (exercise, massage, or a hot bath will increase absorption).

Still, the variability in absorption does not completely account for the day-to-day variability in insulin action observed for human insulin and analogs alike. Studies show that insulin action, regular or analog, can vary as much as 25% for regular insulin and 50% for long acting insulin in the same individual.[450]

Part of the problem may be because insulin excreted by the pancreas normally goes directly to the liver and quickly suppresses that organ's glucose production. About half of this insulin is taken up by the liver and never reaches the general circulation. The concentration of insulin in the portal blood (between the pancreas and liver) is normally four to eight times greater than that in general circulation. This ratio cannot be achieved with injected insulin, which goes directly into the general circulation.

Someday, when everyone has an Internet TV, a videophone, and a robot doing their housework, insulin will no longer be injected, but rather inhaled. Yes, inhaled insulin is just around the corner, but as the joke goes, don't hold your breath. This format is currently only being used for delivery of fast-acting insulin, so some slow-acting insulin will still have to be injected for type 1 diabetics. The action of inhaled insulin is no faster or more consistent than injection and is less efficient, requiring more insulin to achieve the same performance. Moreover, the dosing is less precise than injections. Regarding safety, there is some question as to whether chronic inhalation of a growth hormone will cause any problems, but it is still too early to tell. Annual tests for lung function are recommended for Exubera, the first inhaled insulin product on the market.

Inhaled insulin is just a convenient delivery format, with the key benefit being patient satisfaction and improved quality of life. The inhaler can reduce the number of injections required for type 1s to one per day, and can mean no shots for type 2s who can still produce some insulin. The first generation inhalers are rather large, about the size of a half-yard of beer, but the insulin powder packs should be stable for up to two years at room temperature.

Continuous Subcutaneous Insulin Infusion, better known as "the pump," attempts to mimic more closely a pancreas by providing insulin in a continuous fashion. The pump provides better control, as measured by HbA1c scores, than insulin injections, but current multiple injection therapies using insulin analogs, frequent blood glucose monitoring, and dosage adjustments are nearly as good. Overall, studies show a reduction in HbA1c of about 0.5 for pump users.[451] Pumps are still different from pancreases and similar to injections in that insulin is delivered subcutaneously rather than directly to the liver. Because insulin is absorbed, insulin action is as variable as with needles and hypoglycemia is still a concern.

The implanted insulin pump, also known as the "hockey puck" or "artificial pancreas," addresses some of the limitations of the common insulin pump. Insulin is delivered to the liver first, just as nature intended it, with less variability of action than subcutaneous injection. Blood sugar control, as measured by HbA1c, is as good or better than subcutaneous injection, but with significantly fewer episodes of severe hypoglycemia.[452] The implanted pump is out of site and protected, and is controlled by remote control. The cost of the implant is significantly more than the common pump, but may be worth it in terms of the benefits it provides. Ultimately the choice of delivery method will probably depend on whether one prefers a hockey puck implanted under the skin to a pager worn externally.

The future of insulin pump therapy may lie in systems that dispense insulin in response to measured glucose levels.[453] These feedback-based mechanisms are known as "closed loop" systems. The subcutaneous pump is impractical for closed loop systems due to the slow and variable action of absorbed insulin, but the implanted pump with its direct line to the liver is an ideal candidate. The implanted pump can administer insulin that acts fast enough to respond to feedback from an implanted glucose sensor; however, making this theory a reality—providing a safe, reliable, affordable artificial pancreas—is a challenge that has yet to be met.

Even more challenging has been the task of developing a drug that safely and effectively treats type 2 diabetes. We have a variety of drugs, called oral hypoglycemic agents, that are aimed at lowering blood sugar using various techniques. As we saw in chapter 9, there is plenty of sugarcoating about what these drugs do and how they work. Here is what we really know about each of them.

Pancreas Squeezers (Sulfonylureas)

One way to lower glucose is to get the pancreas to produce more insulin. Scientists have known for many years how to do this. To produce insulin, the beta cells have to work together to create what is called a calcium wave. During a calcium wave, calcium floods into the beta cells causing insulin granules to be secreted out. Just taking lots of calcium doesn't do anything to start the wave. Electricity is what allows minerals like calcium, sodium, and potassium to flow in and out of cells. Calcium can only flow when the voltage across the cell membrane is in a certain range.

Sulfonylureas, let's just call them *SUs*, are drugs that induce insulin secretion by adjusting the cell membrane voltage to induce the flow of calcium. How do they do that? By mimicking the way a healthy body does it. After a meal, glucose levels in the blood are elevated. When the beta cell metabolizes greater amounts of glucose, it blocks the flow of potassium through the beta cell membrane. When potassium flow decreases, the voltage across the membrane changes to favor calcium flow and insulin is released. SUs work by blocking the flow of potassium, which opens the calcium channel and starts the calcium wave. SUs are sometimes referred to as potassium channel blockers. There are other drugs you may have heard of, called calcium channel blockers, that perform the opposite function.

Like *Star Trek*, SUs have different generations. The first generation SUs are about as old as Captain Kirk, and, like actor William Shatner, are hardly used anymore. Like the characters on *Next Generation*, the newer, second generation SUs have interesting names like glyburide (glibenclamide in Europe), glipizide, glicazide, tolazamide, and glimepiride. These are marketed under names such as Amaryl, DiaBeta, Glucotrol, Glynase, and Micronase. Now there are even spinoffs known as

Prandin, Starlix, and Deep Space Nine. More on those in a minute.

SUs do lower blood sugars in some patients and can reduce HbA1c values by a point or more within sixteen weeks of treatment.[454,455] However, studies show that only one in four patients with type 2 diabetes will reach a desired goal of fasting blood sugar < 140 mg/dL using SUs alone, and of those who do succeed initially, there is a failure rate of about five to seven percent per year.[456] After ten years most patients require the addition of some other agent to lower glucose levels. SUs don't work for everybody, and they seldom work alone because they lose their effectiveness over time.

Some have theorized that this is because chronic over-stimulation of the pancreas with SUs causes the beta cells to burn out.[457] However, results from the United Kingdom Prospective Diabetes Study (UKPDS), a clinical trial that monitored 3867 newly diagnosed type 2 diabetics for more than 10 years, showed that the same thing happens with metformin, another oral hypoglycemic agent that does not stimulate the pancreas. In fact, all therapies used in the UKPDS failed similarly to provide long-term blood glucose control. After an initial drop in HbA1c during the first year, HbA1c levels increased at the same rate for all therapies.[458]

Another thing the UKPDS showed is that treatment with SUs is associated with weight gain and higher blood pressure.[459] However, the UKPDS showed no effect, positive or negative, of SUs on heart disease.[460] This was in contrast to the results of another clinical trial, the University Group Diabetes Program (UGDP) study, which showed an increased risk of death from cardiovascular disease in patients taking SUs.[461] As with Rezulin in the Diabetes Prevention Program, the SU arm of the UGDP study was stopped due to the significant increase in number of deaths.

Although the UGDP study has been criticized, SUs now come with the following warning label:

WARNINGS

SPECIAL WARNING ON INCREASED RISK OF CARDIOVASCULAR MORTALITY

The administration of oral hypoglycemic drugs has been reported to be associated with increased cardiovascular mortality as compared to treatment with diet alone or diet plus insulin. This is based on the study conducted by the University Group Diabetes Program (UGDP), a long-term prospective clinical trial designed to evaluate the effectiveness of glucose-lowering drugs in preventing or delaying vascular complications in patients with type 2 diabetes. The study involved 823 patients who were randomly assigned to one of four treatment groups (Diabetes , 19, SUPP. 2: 747-830, 1970).

UGDP reported that patients treated for 5 to 8 years with diet plus a fixed dose of tolbutamide (1.5 grams per day) had a rate of cardiovascular mortality approximately 2½ times that of patients treated with diet alone. A significant increase in total mortality was not observed, but the use of tolbutamide was discontinued based on the increase in cardiovascular mortality, thus limiting the opportunity for the study to show an increase in overall mortality. Despite controversy regarding the interpretation of these results, the findings of the UGDP study provide an adequate basis for this warning. The patient should be informed of the potential Although only one drug in the sulfonylurea class (tolbutamide) was included in this study, it is prudent from a safety standpoint to consider that this warning may also apply to other oral hypoglycemic drugs in this class, in view of their close similarities in mode of action and chemical structure.

Figure C.1: Warnings for sulfonylureas

SUs can cause hypoglycemia because they indiscriminately stimulate insulin secretion, even at low glucose levels. In an attempt to solve this problem, scientists have developed a new class of drugs, known as meglitinide analogs. We'll just call them SU-spinoffs.

These SU spinoffs, marketed as Prandin and Starlix (I was just kidding about the one named Deep Space Nine), are derived from the "non-sulfonylurea" portion of a sulfonylurea. (Yes, you read that right) They work the same way as SUs—they open up calcium channels in beta cells—but they do so by binding to a different site of the sulfonylurea receptor. SU-spinoffs are claimed to be faster acting than regular SUs, providing better insulin secretion after a meal with less stimulation of insulin between meals.

While you will find numerous articles by key opinion leaders explaining how SU-spinoffs provide better post-meal glucose control and result in fewer hypoglycemic episodes than SUs, the evidence to support these claims is lacking. One short-term study found the SU-spinoff had a sooner but lower peak insulin response than the SU, with the same glucose lowering effect.[462] Another found the SU-spinoff worked better than one of two SUs it was tested against, but only in the non-diabetic subjects of the study.[463] (This should come as a great relief to those billions of non-diabetics who have been eagerly awaiting a better SU-spinoff)

A one-year study performed on diabetic subjects found the SU-spinoff "was able to maintain glycaemic control" while "control deteriorated significantly" with the comparison drug, a SU.[464] Yes, we know from studies like the UKPDS that control deteriorates, but only after the first year. Why didn't this six-month study duplicate the amazing first year glucose lowering effects of SUs seen in the UKPDS? Perhaps because the dose of the comparison SU used was 1/8 to 3/8 of the max recommended dosage (*Minification*).

Whether the SU-spinoffs provide any real benefit over existing SUs remains to be seen.

Lilac Extracts (Metformin)

The use of plants in diabetes treatment dates as far back as medieval times, when the French Lilac, known as Goat's Rue, was prescribed to those stricken with relentless urination, the outward symptom of diabetes. The active ingredient in the French Lilac, isoamylene guanidine, does indeed have glucose lowering properties, but when isolated is too toxic to be used for the treatment of diabetes. However, when two guanidine rings are linked, forming a biguanide, the substance can be used safely and effectively. Well, sort of.

The only three lilac extract drugs ever created, metformin, phenformin, and buformin, were all developed in 1957. The latter two enjoyed popularity in the 1960s but were banned after phenformin was associated with cardiovascular disease and lactic acidosis in the UGDP study.[465] Phenformin holds the distinction of being the only drug ever to be forcefully removed by the FDA. Normally, when the FDA asks the manufacturer to withdraw the drug voluntarily, the company complies. However, in an unprecedented move, phenformin's maker, Ceiba-Geigy, objected to the FDA's request defending that patients were dying from other factors. Despite the company's objections, phenformin was taken off the market in 1976 as an imminent hazard.

Metformin has been used in France since 1958, but was not approved for sale in the U.S. until December 1994. Despite the stigma of its evil stepsisters, metformin, marketed as Glucophage, has become a Cinderella story, reaching blockbuster status in the U.S.

Now that generic metformin has come on the market, killing the high-priced exclusivity Glucophage enjoyed for diabetes treatment and now prevention, Glucophage is being pitched as a treatment for polycystic ovary syndrome (PCOS), an aid to weight loss, and an anti-aging product.[466] Remember the story of Neurontin? It will be interesting to see if Bristol-Myers Squibb can find a new market for its pricey Glucophage.

While it is doubtful that metformin will prevent aging there is good evidence that it does help prevent diabetes. The Diabetes Prevention Program, a major clinical trial involving 3,234 people with pre-diabetes, showed that treatment with metformin reduced the risk of getting type 2 diabetes by 31 percent.[467] (Diet and exercise were twice as effective at preventing diabetes in that study).

Metformin is as effective as SUs in reducing blood sugar.[468] A sub-study of the UKPDS involving 1,704 obese, newly diagnosed type 2 diabetics showed that metformin with diet education reduced the mean HbA1c by 0.6% (8.0% versus 7.4%) over diet education alone.[469] However, like SUs, the effectiveness of metformin declines over time. After an initial improvement in the first year, the rate of increase in HbA1c over the course of ten years was the same for drug and non-drug groups in the UKPDS.[470]

Metformin's mechanism of action is not fully understood. What we do know is that metformin appears to make the muscles remove more glucose from the blood and deter the liver from putting glucose into the blood. Thus, it is often stated that metformin improves insulin sensitivity of the muscles and liver. If this is true, it is not clear why. The effect does not happen when metformin is administered intravenously, as opposed to orally.[471] This behavior has led some to believe that metformin works by inhibiting glucose absorption from the gut, rather than by improving insulin sensitivity.

Since metformin does not stimulate insulin secretion, it rarely causes weight gain or hypoglycemia when used by itself. However, like phenformin, metformin has been associated with cases of lactic acidosis.[472] It is not clear how or why this happens, but it is believed that these drugs increase anaerobic metabolism, which creates a buildup of lactic acid. Phenformin does so more actively than metformin and the risk of developing lactic acidosis is 10 to 20 times higher with phenformin than with metformin.[473] While metformin is safer with regard to lactic acidosis, it still carries the legacy of its wicked stepsister with a label warning about lactic acidosis and cardiovascular mortality.

> **WARNING**: A small number of people who have taken GLUCOPHAGE have developed a serious condition called lactic acidosis. Lactic acidosis is caused by a buildup of lactic acid in the blood. This happens more often in people with kidney problems. Most people with kidney problems should not take GLUCOPHAGE or GLUCOPHAGE XR.

> The UGDP reported that patients treated for 5 to 8 years with diet plus a fixed dose of tolbutamide (1.5 g per day) or diet plus a fixed dose of phenformin (100 mg per day), had a rate of cardiovascular mortality approximately 2.5 times that of patients treated with diet alone, resulting in discontinuation of both of these treatments in the UGDP study. Total mortality was increased in both the tolbutamide- and phenformin-treated groups and this increase was statistically significant in the phenformin-treated group. Despite controversy regarding the interpretation of these results, the findings of the UGDP study provide an adequate basis for this warning. The patient should be informed of the potential risks and benefits of metformin HCl and alternative modes of therapy.

Figure C.2: Warnings for metformin

The Carbinators (Alpha-glucosidase inhibitors)

Acarbose (marketed as Precose and Glucobay) and miglitol (marketed as Glyset) make up the class of drugs known as Alpha-glucosidase inhibitors. Let's call them Carbinators, because like *The Terminator*, their job is to terminate the absorption of carbohydrates after a meal. Specifically, carbinators lower blood sugar by slowing down the digestion of carbohydrates after a meal. This happens because the enzyme that breaks medium-sized starches down into glucose has a much greater affinity for the carbinator than it does for starch. Thus, when taken with starchy meals, carbinators can reduce post-meal blood sugar spikes and this ultimately helps reduce fasting blood sugars.

According to published studies, carbinators are as effective as SUs and metformin in lowering post-meal blood glucose levels, but less potent at lowering fasting blood glucose.[474,475]

Carbinators also give you the runs. The most common side effects of carbinators are flatulence, diarrhea, and cramps, which are probably due to the accumulation of undigested carbohydrate in the lower gastrointestinal tract.

High doses of acarbose, one type of carbinator, are associated with elevated liver enzymes and regular monitoring of liver function is recommended for acarbose. Does this sound familiar? However, clinical trial data indicates that miglitol, another type of carbinator, is not associated with elevated liver enzymes.[476] Speaking of elevated liver enzymes ...

The Rezulin Family (Thiazolidinediones)

Rezulin, or troglitazone, was the first of a new class of drugs called thiazolidinediones or TZDs. Just before Rezulin was recalled in March of 2000, pioglitazone (marketed as Actos) and rosiglitazone (marketed as Avandia) came on the U.S. market.

TZDs are claimed to be the first class of medication aimed specifically at improving insulin sensitivity. They appear to improve glucose uptake in the muscles and suppress the liver's production of glucose, but exactly how is unknown. From what we do know about their mechanism of action, it appears to happen indirectly. TZDs bind to receptors that are found in fat tissue, the lower intestine, and immune-related cells, but not in muscle cells. This binding speeds up gene transcription, hastening the production of new fat cells. These new fat cells pull triglycerides and free fatty acids from the blood and secrete a substance called adiponectin (a.k.a. Acrp 30) that is known to inhibit glucose release from the liver and improve insulin sensitivity.[477,478,479] Whatever the mechanism, TZDs decrease both fasting and post meal glucose levels by approximately 20%, about the same as SUs and metformin.[480]

If you guessed that TZDs make you gain weight, you are right. They may also produce other side effects, such as water retention and swelling of the ankles, muscle weakness, and fatigue.[481] Fluid retention is an important concern because it may lead to heart failure. Also of concern are reports of TZD-related congestive heart failure from Canada Health and the Mayo Clinic[482,483] and a study of a health insurance claims database that suggests that TZDs may increase the risk of heart failure.[484]

Like Rezulin, Actos and Avandia require regular liver monitoring, but unlike Rezulin, the monitoring appears to be working. According to one paper published in September of 2004, only eleven cases of TZD-induced liver injury have been reported for Actos and Avandia.[485] In most cases, when the TZD was discontinued, patients improved symptomatically and liver enzyme levels returned to normal within six months.

There have apparently been some fatal adverse reactions to these TZDs. Both TZDs have undergone label changes to reflect risk of liver injury. The following is an excerpt from the Actos label.

WARNINGS

Cardiac Failure and Other Cardiac Effects

ACTOS, like other thiazolidinediones, can cause fluid retention when used alone or in combination with other antidiabetic agents, including insulin. Fluid retention may lead to or exacerbate heart failure. Patients should be observed for signs and symptoms of heart failure (see Information for Patients). ACTOS should be discontinued if any deterioration in cardiac status occurs.

During pre-approval placebo-controlled clinical trials in the U. S., a total of 4 of 1526 (0.26%) patients treated with ACTOS and 2 of 793 (0.25%) placebo-treated patients had ALT values 3 times the upper limit of normal. The ALT elevations in patients treated with ACTOS were reversible and were not clearly related to therapy with ACTOS. In postmarketing experience with ACTOS, reports of hepatitis and of hepatic enzyme elevations to 3 or more times the upper limit of normal have been received. Very rarely, these reports have involved hepatic failure with and without fatal outcome, although causality has not been established.

Figure C.3: Warnings for Actos

It remains to be seen whether any of Rezulin's cousins are safe or effective over time.

Byetta (Exenatide)

Exenatide is the first in a new class of medicines known as incretin mimetics under investigation for the treatment of type 2 diabetes. In clinical trials, exenatide has demonstrated reductions in blood sugar and improvements in markers of beta cell function. Islet regeneration therapy appears to be a promising line of research. Many are investigating the properties of Glucagon-like Peptide 1 (GLP-1), a hormone that most type 2 diabetics are deficient in, has been shown to reverse the negative cycle of diabetes.[486] GLP-1 is a superstar hormone that stimulates insulin production, prevents beta cell destruction, and facilitates growth of new beta cells.[487,488,489]

Until recently, GLP-1 had not received much attention because, having a half-life in the blood of a few minutes, it was not attractive to drug companies. But that all changed when endocrinologist Dr. John Eng encountered the endangered Gila Monster of the American southwest and northern Mexico. In Mexico, where Gila Monsters must go for long periods without food, these lizards have developed the ability to keep their insulin low and then spike it when food comes around. The Gila Monster is one of only two venomous lizards in the world. Its venom, Eng discovered, contains a protein that is similar in structure to GLP-1 and has a plasma half-life of twelve hours. Eng named this protein extendin, and has licensed a patent for it to a pharmaceutical company that is now producing it synthetically (they're not running around Mexico slurping saliva from endangered Gila Monsters).

Recently there have been other pharmaceutical companies

interested in developing GLP-1-like treatments. This is very promising because GLP-1 therapies target the cause of the disease rather than the symptoms, as today's clinical treatments do. Treatments that address beta-cell destruction could represent a significant new development in the management of type 2 diabetes, since they may actually reverse the disease.

Future Drugs for Diabetes

The Cure for Diabetes may lie, of all places, in a cigarette carton. Specifically, the cellophane wrapping from Imperial Tobacco, Montreal Canada, is the stuff used in the lab of Dr. Aaron I. Vinik. In 1983, Dr. Vinik and colleague, Dr. Lawrence Rosenberg, wrapped a hamster pancreas in cellophane to examine the inflammatory processes of pancreatic disease. They were surprised to find that instead of inducing inflammation, the pancreases bound in cellophane were growing new islet cells. With further experiments, they showed that diabetes could be reversed in hamsters (50% of them) by wrapping the head of the pancreas with cigarette package covering.[490]

This was exciting news. If the scientists could isolate the substance that was causing the growth of new islet cells, perhaps it could be used to naturally repair the damaged pancreases of type 1 and type 2 diabetics. It was soon discovered that Ilotropin was the element in the cellophane that stimulated cell growth. For years Dr. Vinik and colleagues tried to isolate a pure form of Ilotropin, but it proved challenging. Frustrated, they decided to take a different path. Aided by the work of the human genome project they began to search for the gene that initiated the creation of Ilotropin and new islet cells. In 1997 they discovered such a gene, which they named Islet Neogenesis Associated Protein, or INGAP.

When INGAP was given to normal animals they developed an

increase in their beta cell mass but did not over secrete insulin and never became hypoglycemic. The researchers believe that this natural balance occurred due to transcription factor PDX, the mechanism that prevents the overproduction of new cells by down regulating the INGAP gene.

In April 1997, a month before the discovery of INGAP was to be published, pharmaceutical giant Lilly signed a licensing agreement with the discovering universities to develop and commercialize this novel approach to treat and possibly cure diabetes. However, two years later Lilly decided to stop funding INGAP research. According to Lilly it was not because INGAP wasn't promising, but because it wasn't a good business model.[491] (Example of a good business model: Lilly generates over two billion dollars a year from its line of insulins and other diabetes products, all of which are designed for lifetime use.)

Undeterred, Vinik and associates continued animal and test tube studies. In the spring of 2001 INGAP was picked up by GMP Companies and human clinical trials began later that year. Proctor and Gamble Pharmaceuticals joined the venture in 2002. The phase 1 trials have found INGAP to be safe in humans, and phase 2 clinical trials are now underway to determine whether it is effective.

If successful, INGAP would represent a shift in the treatment of diabetes from addressing the symptoms, to addressing the problem, and ultimately reversing the disease. If INGAP can stimulate enough beta cell growth to overcome antibodies, it may be a natural cure for type 1 diabetes. However, it may be more effective for treating type 2 diabetes, where the rate of beta cell loss is much slower.

The sixty-four thousand dollar question is does INGAP cure

diabetes in humans? In human clinical trials, INGAP increased C-peptide levels in type 1 and type 2 diabetic patients, indicating that new islets were being formed. A modest 0.6 percent drop in HbA1c was observed in type 2 diabetics.[492]

After the clinical trials the license for INGAP was dropped by Proctor & Gamble and picked up by newly formed Kinexum Metabolics Inc. Dr. G. Alexander Fleming, President and CEO of Kinexum, believes that INGAP Peptide "offers excellent prospects for a breakthrough therapy and the achievement of a major scientific milestone."[493] Fleming was formerly the Food and Drug Administration's senior endocrinologist and clinical group leader for the evaluation and regulation of diabetes and metabolic therapies. He is also the man who "eased out" John Gueriguian and his report so that Rezulin could be approved. Although Fleming & Co. consider the INGAP Peptide to be Kinexum's "lead compound," the word INGAP is not mentioned anywhere on Kinexum's website.[494]

Whether or not INGAP will ever become a treatment for diabetes, beta cell regeneration is a promising line of research. In addition to INGAP, other substances, such as gastrin, Epidermal Growth Factor (EGF), and GLP-1 (the protein from the Gila Monster), that also promote beta cell growth are being actively explored by a number of pharmaceutical companies.

Appendix D—The HELP Principle

This appendix describes how the principle of HELP—*High Essentials / Lighter Portions*—applies to various types of foods. As you know, there are a number of essential vitamins and minerals, fatty acids, and amino acids that our body must get from diet (See Table D.1)

Essential Vitamins	vitamin A, vitamin C, vitamin D, vitamin E, vitamin K, thiamine (B1), riboflavin (B2), niacin (B3), pyridoxine (B6), folate, cyanocobalamine (B12), biotin, and pantothenic acid
Essential Minerals	calcium, phosphorous, magnesium, sodium, chloride, potassium, iron, zinc, iodine, selenium, copper, manganese, chromium, molybdenum, fluorine, and sulfur
Essential Amino Acids	histidine, isoleucine, leucine, lysine, methionine, phenylalanine, threonine, tryptophan, valine
Essential Fatty Acids	linoleic acid, alpha-linolenic acid

Table D.1 Essential vitamins, minerals, amino acids, and fatty acids

In addition to these, there are dozens of other nutrients contained in foods that our bodies need. To get enough of them all we must eat a large variety and amount of food every day. The following sections describe the various families of foods and how they fit into the HELP plan.

Vegetables

Vegetables are the best foods. They have been around for millions of years and are the most nutrient dense foods on the planet. The best natural sources of fiber, vitamin A, vitamin E, vitamin K, folate, vitamin B6, potassium, magnesium, calcium, manganese, and iron are vegetables.

Vegetables have the highest nutrient density when eaten raw or steamed. Ketchup is not a vegetable (sorry Mr. Reagan). Similarly, French fries, spinach casserole, candied yams and other vegetables diluted with empty calories don't qualify as nutrient blockbusters. However, a little butter on your steamed vegetables or dressing on your salad won't totally blow the nutrient density of these high-octane foods. If stir-frying (using pure-pressed, extra virgin olive oil of course) encourages you to eat vegetables, go for it. Just know the difference between adding a few extra calories and creating a food that is more empty calories than it is vegetable. Wash your vegetables, whether they are organic or conventional, as all vegetables contain some amount of pesticides.

Fruits

Fruits have been around for millions of years and provide a variety of nutrients such as fiber, vitamin C, potassium, and manganese. The often-used term "fruits and vegetables" is misleading in putting these two in the same category because fruits are not in the same league as vegetables. Spinach contains six times as much potassium per calorie as a banana and broccoli nearly three times as much vitamin C as an orange. Whereas vegetables generally contain good amounts of essential amino acids and fats, fruits are typically ninety percent or more carbohydrate and mostly sugar.

Because of all the empty calories from sugar, fruits in their raw form are only moderately nutritious. Sugar added forms, such as juices, jellies, canned fruits, fruit cocktail, applesauce, and apple pie are not nutritious choices and will have a dramatic effect on blood sugar even in moderate proportions. Even juices without sugar added raise blood sugar rapidly because juicing removes the fiber that slows absorption and the juice format makes it much easier to consume more sugar calories. Fruits are considered healthy, and rightfully so, but you have to be more careful with them than vegetables. Small portions of raw fruit are the way to go.

Nuts and Seeds

Nuts and seeds provide a wide range of nutrients including protein, essential fatty acids, fiber, and vitamins and minerals. Mixed nuts are a good source of vitamin E, vitamin K, thiamine, niacin, vitamin B6, folate, pantothenic acid, magnesium, manganese, selenium, phosphorous, iron, and copper. No one nut or seed provides high levels of all of these but they each have their own strong suits. When you combine various types of nuts and seeds, you get a tasty mixture that provides a wide variety of essentials.

Nuts and seeds are a great source of unsaturated fatty acids. Fats make up seventy to ninety percent of calories, and most of them are unsaturated. When you eat raw nuts and seeds (i.e., not dry roasted) you get the fats in their natural unprocessed forms. Except for walnuts, almost all nuts have high levels of omega-6 fats, which, according to some dieticians, must be balanced by consumption of foods or supplements rich in omega-3 fatty acids. Adding milled flaxseed to your diet and/or consuming cold-pressed flaxseed oil will improve the ratio, as flaxseeds are the richest source of essential omega-3 fatty acids on the planet.

Nuts and seeds pack a lot of calories, so they cannot afford to carry extra empty calories, as in honey roasted peanuts, beer nuts, sugar-added peanut butter, and peanut M&Ms. Prefer them in raw form and forget about getting the nutrition from sugar-free peanut butter cups.

Nuts and seeds typically contain about fifteen percent protein and fifteen percent carbohydrates. Because a nut/seed mix provides such a wide array of nutrients and is convenient to transport it makes an ideal snack food. Consumption of nuts and peanut butter is correlated with a reduced risk of type 2 diabetes.[495]

Whole Grains

Whole grain foods contain all three parts of the grain: bran, germ, and endosperm. Together these three are a good source of thiamin, riboflavin, niacin, vitamin B6, folate, vitamin E, selenium, zinc, copper, magnesium, selenium, manganese, and fiber.

Unfortunately, the vast majority of grain products on the market are made from refined flour, the fiberless and nutrient-poor scrap left over from the pulverization of whole grains. Most so-called whole wheat bread is made from enriched refined flour with bran added back to it and molasses for coloring. These breads are not whole grain. Real whole grain products are hard to find because food labels are notoriously misleading. The terms "wheat," "wheat flour," "multi-grain," "oat bran," "seven-grain," "nine-grain," "stoned wheat," "wheatberry," and "whole bran" are often used to describe non-whole grain breads. The phrase "made with whole grain" often means, "Yes, we put one actual whole grain in, but along with 99% refined flour." Sadly, the word "whole," which perfectly sums up how we should eat our foods, has become an overused marketing term, resulting in meaningless, but healthy sounding words like "wholesome," which is used to make chocolate cream-filled cup cakes sound healthy.

To find real whole grain products, check the ingredients. Look for sprouted or cracked whole wheat. Make sure enriched wheat flour is not the first or second ingredient listed. Check the fiber content. While high fiber is not a sufficient condition to determine that a product is whole grain, it is a necessary one. Make sure there aren't any added calories in the form of sugar or partially hydrogenated vegetable oils.

Grains are not as nutritionally dense as vegetables or fruits, so there is not much room for caloric dilution. Some natural peanut butter on toast is an acceptable choice as it adds nutrients with the calories. Finally, moderate your portion sizes. Whole grain foods often contain plenty of carbohydrates and will raise blood sugar levels. Use your meter to determine how much you can handle.

Meat

Beef, lamb, pork, poultry, and other game all fall under the category of meat. Meats are high in protein, thiamin, niacin, vitamin B6, vitamin B12, phosphorus, selenium, and zinc. If you like liver, it provides an even greater assortment of essentials.

When selecting meat you should be able to identify the animal it came from and which part of the animal. "Ambiguous" meats such as sausages, chicken nuggets, salami and luncheon loaf generally have fewer essential nutrients per calorie than a steak, chicken breast, pork chop, or leg of lamb. The probability of bacterial infection is much greater in ground beef, which may come from the meat of thousands of cows, than in a steak that comes from a single cow.

Meat grilled with spices is one of life's truly great pleasures and has fewer empty calories than meat lathered in sugary barbeque sauce or battered and fried in trans fatty acids. Organic grass fed beef is more expensive than industrial beef, but it provides more omega-3 fatty acids and, by law, should not contain hormones or antibiotics.

Seafood

The sea provides us with a plethora of foods that are high in essentials. Fish are an excellent source of protein and essential fatty acids. They are chock full of essential vitamins and minerals such as vitamin D, thiamin, niacin, vitamin B6, vitamin B12. Other sea creatures such as shrimp, crab, lobster, oysters, clams, and mussels can be good sources of protein, vitamin C, thiamin, riboflavin, niacin, vitamin B12, folate, magnesium, potassium, phosphorus, zinc, copper, iron, manganese, and selenium.

Unfortunately most seafood is contaminated with unsafe levels of mercury. As of May 2006, the most contaminated are shark, swordfish, king mackerel, tilefish, tuna steaks, canned tuna, largemouth bass, sea bass, gulf coast oysters, marlin, halibut, walleye, white croaker, and pike. The least contaminated are mid-Atlantic blue crab, croaker, fish sticks, summer flounder, haddock, farmed trout, and wild Pacific salmon. Most fish oil supplements are safe because they are distilled, which removes mercury. For an up to date list of which fish are most/least contaminated, see the Environmental Working Group's fish list at www.ewg.org/reports/BrainFood/sidebar.html.

Salmon is relatively uncontaminated by mercury, and has become quite a popular fish because it is high in healthy omega-3 fatty acids. One study found farm-raised salmon to contain ten times more toxins than wild caught salmon.[496] However, the farm industry points out that these levels are still well below the FDA standard and that farmers have already taken measures to reduce the amount of toxins and antibiotics fed to fish. Because of their diets, farm raised salmon are naturally gray rather than pink and are fed artificial coloring to make them look more pink like their wild counterparts. It is a common misperception that wild caught salmon contains more omega-3 fatty acids than farm-raised salmon. In fact, there is more variation in omega-3 fatty acid content between different species of salmon than there is between wild and farm-raised salmon of the same species. Farmed Atlantic salmon actually has a higher omega-3 fatty acid content than most species of wild salmon.

Fish and other seafood are great carbohydrate-free sources of essentials when they are not breaded and fried. Battering and frying adds empty calories and often trans fatty acids to an otherwise healthy food. So when we talk about healthy seafood, we are not talking about fish filets, fish sticks, or any part of the Red Lobster Admiral's Feast. Little crunchy goldfish don't count either.

Legumes

Legumes include beans, lentils, tempeh, tofu, chickpeas, soybeans, and any other food that ends in the word "beans" (except string beans, green beans, and jelly beans). All legumes are excellent sources of fiber and protein. They are high in vitamins, such as folate and thiamin, and minerals such as zinc, copper, magnesium iron, phosphorous, potassium, and manganese.

In their natural form or cooked in water legumes provide many essentials per calorie. Barbeque baked beans contain empty calories from sugar and refried beans from fat but the amounts vary so check the product labels. Use your glucometer to determine which products and what portion sizes are appropriate for you.

Dairy

Dairy products like milk, cheeses, and yogurt provide protein, riboflavin, vitamin B12, vitamin D, calcium, potassium, phosphorus, and zinc. However, these nutrients always come packaged with significant amounts of sugar and/or fat. Even low fat and nonfat versions, which don't taste as creamy, are nutritionally dilute. For example, when you get your recommended daily allowance of calcium from three glasses of skim milk you also get about 45 grams of sugar. A daily supply from fat-free, fruit on the bottom yogurt comes with 130 grams of sugar. Cheeses, which have little to no carbohydrates, are a better choice for keeping blood sugar under control, but they contain empty calories in the form of fat. The low fat and nonfat versions of cheese are some of the best ways to get calcium. One cup of low fat Swiss cheese provides 100% of the RDA for calcium, and 32 grams of protein with only 6 grams of fat and 4 grams of carbs.

Aside from containing extra calories from sugar, there are additional concerns about dairy products from the U.S. Cow's milk frequently contains hormones, pesticides and antibiotics, and has been linked to allergies.[497,498] Organic milk is free of these contaminants but it is still pasteurized to remove germs and homogenized to keep the cream evenly distributed. Some believe that these processes destroy the nutrients and denature the proteins, resulting in a nutritionally inferior product to raw milk.[499,500,501]

Milk is not a nutritional superstar, but it is heavily marketed (*got milk?*) by superstars alongside a campaign to induce fear that Americans aren't getting enough calcium and may suffer osteoporosis. As Walter Willett points out in the *Harvard Healthy Eating Guide*, there is no calcium emergency. Americans consume more calcium than most nations and the results from seven long-term prospective studies that have followed large groups of people for several years don't show any important reduction in risk of broken bones with increasing calcium intake. Much of the world is unable to digest lactose, the sugar in dairy, and they get along fine on vegetables such as spinach, argula, and Chinese cabbage, which have more calcium per calorie than any dairy product.

Eggs

Eggs are little oval bundles of nutrients. They are often called the perfect source of protein; their amino acid content and digestibility are the reference against which all other proteins are measured. Moreover, eggs are a good source of riboflavin, vitamin B12, phosphorus, selenium, and, depending on how the hens are fed, omega-3 fatty acids.

The first thing most people have been conditioned to associate with eggs is cholesterol. Eggs contain a lot of cholesterol, but, as we've seen, the "dietary cholesterol causes heart attacks" theory is unfounded. A 1999 study found no evidence of an association between egg consumption and risk of CHD or stroke in healthy men and women. There was a weak association for those with diabetes, which warrants further research.[502]

Nowadays eggs are marketed as heart healthy. They contain healthy carotenoids such as lutein and zeaxanthin and egg manufacturers are now producing "designer" eggs lower in cholesterol and higher in healthy fats. Hens fed diets high in vitamin E and omega-3 fatty acids produce eggs with high vitamin E and omega-3 fatty acid content in the yolks. Cage-free, free-range, and organic eggs are nutritionally similar to regular eggs if the feed is of the same quality. Egg creams and Eggo waffles are not as healthy as eggs.

Drinks

Water is the king of drinks. It is one hundred percent essential to the human body and contains no calories. If you like the taste of your tap water, it is an economical source. Bottled spring water and mineral water are purer sources that contain a number of trace minerals. If it doesn't say "spring water" on the label, it probably came from a tap. *Dasani* and *Aquafina* are just filtered municipal water from Coke and Pepsi respectively. You don't need to drink eight 8-ounce glasses a day—this is an oversimplified urban legend. You need to drink as much as your body needs, which varies greatly depending on the environment, what type of food you eat, and your activity level. A number of vitamin-added waters are available and these are fine, but if you have decided you need supplementation, there are less expensive ways to get it than by drinking vitamin water.

Antioxidants and small amounts of other vitamins can be found in tea (especially green tea) and coffee, which are also virtually calorie free if you don't add milk and sugar. Caffeine has been shown to decrease insulin sensitivity and impair glucose tolerance.[503,504,505] However, a recent study in the Netherlands showed that people who drank at least seven cups of coffee a day were half as likely to develop type 2 diabetes mellitus as people who drank 2 cups or less a day.[506] Other studies have confirmed that risk decreases with more coffee and that, while the association holds for regular and decaffeinated coffee, it is stronger for regular coffee. [507,508,509]

The high-fructose corn syrup family of drinks like sodas, sports drinks, energy drinks, fake juices, and essentially anything whose name ends with the word "drink" provide little or no nutritional value with lots of empty calories in the form of sugar.

Juices, wine, and beer provide small amounts of essential vitamins and minerals along with plenty of empty calories. Although the nutritional value of these drinks is touted by winemakers and the like, you are not going to drink your way to healthy nutrition; not without the side effects of massive amounts of calories, sugar and/or alcohol. Spirits straight up or on the rocks are the lowest carbohydrate forms of alcohol, but they still contain calories. Most mixers for drinks, such as margarita mix, tonic, etc. are loaded with sugar.

For all its empty calories alcohol has some beneficial effects for diabetics. While the liver is busy processing alcohol it produces less glucose and stores less glycogen. As the liver runs out of glycogen, its cells become more sensitive to insulin. Moderate alcohol consumption has been shown to improve insulin sensitivity and is associated with a decreased incidence of diabetes mellitus and heart disease in persons with diabetes.[510,511,512] However, these effects reverse with heavy consumption (greater than three drinks per day).[513,514] The consensus on alcohol is that for optimal health it should be drunk in moderation. Moderation means one drink per day per 100 lbs of body weight. Gaining weight to increase your quota is not a good idea.

Miscellaneous

The inner aisles of the supermarket are filled with products that are marketed as foods but are really nutrient depleted items that have been invented in the last 100 years. The top three ingredients are invariably sugar, flour, and partially hydrogenated vegetable oil. You can find low fat and sugar-free versions of these products, but, as we have learned, taking out one ingredient doesn't magically make a junk food healthy. Rather than call them "food," these products should be considered entertainment. All entertainment has a price, and these products carry a cost to your health. Remember this when choosing to treat yourself. When the occasion merits it treat yourself well, but do so in moderation.

Appendix E—Recommended Reading

There are many excellent books related to diabetes management. The following is a short list of some of the best.

Dr. Bernstein's Diabetes Solution: A Complete Guide to Achieving Normal Blood Sugars by Richard K. Bernstein. Little, Brown; 1st ed edition (May, 1997) ISBN: 0316093440

The Schwarzbein Principle: The Truth About Losing Weight, Being Healthy, and Feeling Younger by Diana Schwarzbein, Nancy Deville. HCI (May 1, 1999) ISBN: 1558746803

Eat, Drink, and Be Healthy: The Harvard Medical School Guide to Healthy Eating by Walter C. Willett, P. J. Skerrett. Free Press (July 30, 2002). ISBN: 0743223225

Know Your Fats: The Complete Primer for Understanding the Nutrition of Fats, Oils and Cholesterol by Mary G. Enig. Bethesda Press (May 14, 2000) ISBN: 0967812607

Index

References

[1] Diabetes Prevention Research Group: Reduction in the evidence of type 2 diabetes with life-style intervention or metformin. New England Journal of Medicine 346:393-403, 2002.

[2] Lindstrom J, Louheranta A, Mannelin M, Rastas M, Salminen V, Eriksson J, Uusitupa M, Tuomilehto J; Finnish Diabetes Prevention Study Group. The Finnish Diabetes Prevention Study (DPS): Lifestyle intervention and 3-year results on diet and physical activity. Diabetes Care. 2003 Dec;26(12):3230-6.

[3] Pan XR, Li GW, Hu YH, Wang JX, Yang WY, An ZX, Hu ZX, Lin J, Xiao JZ, Cao HB, Liu PA, Jiang XG, Jiang YY, Wang JP, Zheng H, Zhang H, Bennett PH, Howard BV. Effects of diet and exercise in preventing NIDDM in people with impaired glucose tolerance. The Da Qing IGT and Diabetes Study. Diabetes Care. 1997 Apr;20(4):537-44.

[4] Enig, "Know Your Fats: The Complete Primer for Understanding the Nutrition of Fats, Oils and Cholesterol", Bethesda Press, 14 May, 2000.

[5] Young CM, Scanlan SS, Im HS, Lutwak L. Effect of body composition and other parameters in obese young men of carbohydrate level of reduction diet. Am J Clin Nutr. 1971 Mar;24(3):290-6.

[6] Rabast U, Schonborn J, Kasper H. Dietetic treatment of obesity with low and high-carbohydrate diets: comparative studies and clinical results. Int J Obes. 1979;3(3):201-11.

[7] Lean ME, Han TS, Prvan T, Richmond PR, Avenell A. Weight loss with high and low carbohydrate 1200 kcal diets in free living women.Eur J Clin Nutr. 1997 Apr;51(4):243-8.

[8] Skov AR, Toubro S, Ronn B, Holm L, Astrup A.Randomized trial on protein vs carbohydrate in ad libitum fat reduced diet for the treatment of obesity. Int J Obes Relat Metab Disord. 1999 May;23(5):528-36.

[9] Willi SM, Oexmann MJ, Wright NM, Collop NA, Key LL Jr.The effects of a high-protein, low-fat, ketogenic diet on adolescents with morbid obesity: body composition, blood chemistries, and sleep abnormalities. Pediatrics. 1998

Jan;101(1 Pt 1):61-7.

[10] Sharman MJ, Gomez AL, Kraemer WJ, Volek JS.Very low-carbohydrate and low-fat diets affect fasting lipids and postprandial lipemia differently in overweight men. J Nutr. 2004 Apr;134(4):880-5.

[11] Garrow JS, Summerbell CD.Meta-analysis: effect of exercise, with or without dieting, on the body composition of overweight subjects. Eur J Clin Nutr. 1995 Jan;49(1):1-10.

[12] Benoit FL, Martin RL, Watten RH. Changes in body composition during weight reduction in obesity. Balance studies comparing effects of fasting and a ketogenic diet. Ann Intern Med. 1965 Oct;63(4):604-12.

[13] Greene, P., Willett, W., Devecis, J., et al., "Pilot 12-Week Feeding Weight-Loss Comparison: Low-Fat vs Low-Carbohydrate (Ketogenic) Diets," Abstract Presented at The North American Association for the Study of Obesity Annual Meeting 2003, Obesity Research, 11S, 2003, page 95OR.

[14] http://atkins.com/Archive/2003/12/22-370922.html

[15] Sondike SB, Copperman N, Jacobson MS. Effects of a low-carbohydrate diet on weight loss and cardiovascular risk factor in overweight adolescents. J Pediatr. 2003 Mar;142(3):253-8.

[16] Sharman MJ, Kraemer WJ, Love DM, Avery NG, Gomez AL, Scheett TP, Volek JS. A ketogenic diet favorably affects serum biomarkers for cardiovascular disease in normal-weight men. J Nutr. 2002 Jul;132(7):1879-85.]

[17] Westman EC, Yancy WS, Edman JS, Tomlin KF, Perkins CE. Effect of 6-month adherence to a very low carbohydrate diet program. Am J Med. 2002 Jul;113(1):30-6.

[18] Foster GD, Wyatt HR, Hill JO, McGuckin BG, Brill C, Mohammed BS, Szapary PO, Rader DJ, Edman JS, Klein S. A randomized trial of a low-carbohydrate diet for obesity. N Engl J Med. 2003 May 22;348(21):2082-90.

[19] Samaha FF, Iqbal N, Seshadri P, Chicano KL, Daily DA, McGrory J, Williams T, Williams M, Gracely EJ, Stern L. A low-carbohydrate as compared with a low-fat diet in severe obesity. N Engl J Med. 2003 May 22;348(21):2074-81.

[20] Yancy WS Jr, Olsen MK, Guyton JR, Bakst RP, Westman EC. A low-carbohydrate, ketogenic diet versus a low-fat diet to treat obesity and hyperlipidemia: a randomized, controlled trial. Ann Intern Med. 2004 May

18;140(10):769-77.

[21] Sharman MJ, Kraemer WJ, Love DM, Avery NG, Gomez AL, Scheett TP, Volek JS. A ketogenic diet favorably affects serum biomarkers for cardiovascular disease in normal-weight men. J Nutr. 2002 Jul;132(7):1879-85.

[22] Larosa JC, Fry AG, Muesing R, Rosing DR.Effects of high-protein, low-carbohydrate dieting on plasma lipoproteins and body weight. J Am Diet Assoc. 1980 Sep;77(3):264-70.

[23] Low CC, Grossman EB, Gumbiner B. Potentiation of effects of weight loss by monounsaturated fatty acids in obese NIDDM patients. Diabetes. 1996 May;45(5):569-75.

[24] Licata A. A., Bou E., Bartter F. C., West F. Acute effects of dietary protein on calcium metabolism in patients with osteoporosis. J. Gerontol. 1981; 36:14-19

[25] Moriguti JC, Ferriolli E, Marchini JS. Urinary calcium loss in elderly men on a vegetable:animal (1:1) high-protein diet. Gerontology. 1999 Sep-Oct;45(5):274-8.

[26] Roughead ZK, Johnson LK, Lykken GI, Hunt JR. Controlled high meat diets do not affect calcium retention or indices of bone status in healthy postmenopausal women.J Nutr. 2003 Apr;133(4):1020-6.

[27] Munger RG, Cerhan JR, Chiu BC. Prospective study of dietary protein intake and risk of hip fracture in postmenopausal women. Am J Clin Nutr. 1999 Jan;69(1):147-52.

[28] Atkins, RC. Dr. Atkins New Diet Revolution. 1st edition. Pg 100. New York: Avon; 1992.

[29] Stern L, Iqbal N, Seshadri P, Chicano KL, Daily DA, McGrory J, Williams M, Gracely EJ, Samaha FF. The effects of low-carbohydrate versus conventional weight loss diets in severely obese adults: one-year follow-up of a randomized trial. Ann Intern Med. 2004 May 18;140(10):778-85.

[30] Gutierrez M, Akhavan M, Jovanovic L, Peterson CM. Utility of a short-term 25% carbohydrate diet on improving glycemic control in type 2 diabetes mellitus. J Am Coll Nutr. 1998 Dec;17(6):595-600.

[31] Parillo M, Giacco R, Ciardullo AV, Rivellese AA, Riccardi G. Does a high-carbohydrate diet have different effects in NIDDM patients treated with diet alone or hypoglycemic drugs? Diabetes Care. 1996 May;19(5):498-500.

[32] Sharman MJ, Gomez AL, Kraemer WJ, Volek JS. Very low-carbohydrate and low-fat diets affect fasting lipids and postprandial lipemia differently in overweight men. J Nutr. 2004 Apr;134(4):880-5.

[33] Volek JS, Sharman MJ, Gomez AL, DiPasquale C, Roti M, Pumerantz A, Kraemer WJ. Comparison of a very low-carbohydrate and low-fat diet on fasting lipids, LDL subclasses, insulin resistance, and postprandial lipemic responses in overweight women. J Am Coll Nutr. 2004 Apr;23(2):177-84.

[34] Nielsen JV, Jonsson E, Nilsson AK. Lasting improvement of hyperglycaemia and bodyweight: low-carbohydrate diet in type 2 diabetes--a brief report. Ups J Med Sci. 2005;110(1):69-73.

[35] Boden G, Sargrad K, Homko C, Mozzoli M, Stein TP. Effect of a low-carbohydrate diet on appetite, blood glucose levels, and insulin resistance in obese patients with type 2 diabetes.Ann Intern Med. 2005 Mar 15;142(6):403-11.

[36] Bernstein RK. Dr. Bernstein's Diabetes Solution: A Complete Guide to Achieving Normal Blood Sugars Little Brown&Company; 1997. ISBN: 0316093440

[37] Ornish D, Brown SE, Scherwitz LW, Billings JH, Armstrong WT, Ports TA, McLanahan SM, Kirkeeide RL, Brand RJ, Gould KL. Can lifestyle changes reverse coronary heart disease? The Lifestyle Heart Trial. Lancet. 1990 Jul 21;336(8708):129-33.

[38] Tuomilehto J, Lindstrom J, Eriksson JG, Valle TT, Hamalainen H, Ilanne-Parikka P, Keinanen-Kiukaanniemi S, Laakso M, Louheranta A, Rastas M, Salminen V, Uusitupa M; Finnish Diabetes Prevention Study Group. Prevention of type 2 diabetes mellitus by changes in lifestyle among subjects with impaired glucose tolerance. N Engl J Med. 2001 May 3;344(18):1343-50.

[39] Knowler WC, Barrett-Connor E, Fowler SE, Hamman RF, Lachin JM, Walker EA, Nathan DM; Diabetes Prevention Program Research Group. Reduction in the incidence of type 2 diabetes with lifestyle intervention or metformin.N Engl J Med. 2002 Feb 7;346(6):393-403.

[40] Pan XR, Li GW, Hu YH, Wang JX, Yang WY, An ZX, Hu ZX, Lin J, Xiao JZ, Cao HB, Liu PA, Jiang XG, Jiang YY, Wang JP, Zheng H, Zhang H, Bennett PH, Howard BV. Effects of diet and exercise in preventing NIDDM in people with impaired glucose tolerance. The Da Qing IGT and Diabetes Study.

Diabetes Care. 1997 Apr;20(4):537-44.

[41] Ornish D, Brown SE, Scherwitz LW, Billings JH, Armstrong WT, Ports TA, McLanahan SM, Kirkeeide RL, Brand RJ, Gould KL. Can lifestyle changes reverse coronary heart disease? The Lifestyle Heart Trial. Lancet. 1990 Jul 21;336(8708):129-33.

[42] Ornish D. Dr. Dean Ornish's Program for Reversing Heart Disease. New York: Random House, 1990; Ballantine Books, 1992.

[43] Sondike SB, Copperman N, Jacobson MS. Effects of a low-carbohydrate diet on weight loss and cardiovascular risk factor in overweight adolescents. J Pediatr. 2003 Mar;142(3):253-8.

[44] Kasper H, Thiel H, Ehl M. Response of body weight to a low carbohydrate, high fat diet in normal and obese subjects. Am J Clin Nutr. 1973 Feb;26(2):197-204.

[45] Westman EC, Yancy WS, Edman JS, Tomlin KF, Perkins CE. Effect of 6-month adherence to a very low carbohydrate diet program. Am J Med. 2002 Jul;113(1):30-6.

[46] Foster GD, Wyatt HR, Hill JO, McGuckin BG, Brill C, Mohammed BS, Szapary PO, Rader DJ, Edman JS, Klein S. A randomized trial of a low-carbohydrate diet for obesity. N Engl J Med. 2003 May 22;348(21):2082-90.

[47] Samaha FF, Iqbal N, Seshadri P, Chicano KL, Daily DA, McGrory J, Williams T, Williams M, Gracely EJ, Stern L. A low-carbohydrate as compared with a low-fat diet in severe obesity. N Engl J Med. 2003 May 22;348(21):2074-81.

[48] Brehm BJ, Seeley RJ, Daniels SR, D'Alessio DA. A randomized trial comparing a very low carbohydrate diet and a calorie-restricted low fat diet on body weight and cardiovascular risk factors in healthy women. J Clin Endocrinol Metab. 2003 Apr;88(4):1617-23.

[49] Yancy WS Jr, Olsen MK, Guyton JR, Bakst RP, Westman EC. A low-carbohydrate, ketogenic diet versus a low-fat diet to treat obesity and hyperlipidemia: a randomized, controlled trial. Ann Intern Med. 2004 May 18;140(10):769-77.

[50] Ornish D. Dr. Dean Ornish's Program for Reversing Heart Disease. New York: Random House, 1990; Ballantine Books, 1992.

[51] Ornish D. Dr. Dean Ornish's Program for Reversing Heart Disease. New

York: Random House, 1990; Ballantine Books, 1992. p 256, 280

[52] Ornish describes his switch to recommending fish oil on WebMD.com. http://my.webmd.com/content/pages/2/3079_1700.htm

[53] Keys, A. Coronary Heart Disease In Seven Countries. Circulation, 41, suppl. 1, 1-211, 1970.

[54] Hu FB. The Mediterranean diet and mortality - olive oil and beyond. N Engl J Med. 2003;348 (26):2595-2596.

[55] Kok FJ, Kromhout D. Atherosclerosis Epidemiological studies on the health effects of a Mediterranean diet. Eur J Nutr. 2004 Mar;43 Suppl 1:I2-I5.

[56] Assmann G, Wahrburg, U. Scientific Evidence for Olive Oil, the Cardiovascular Risk Factors and Coronary Heart Disease. http://www.olivissimo.com/evidence-olive-oil-effects-lipid-metabolism.php

[57] Mensink RP, Katan MB. Effect of a dietary fatty acids on serum lipids and lipoproteins - A meta-analysis of 27 trials. Arteriosclerosis Thromb 12: 911-919 (1992)

[58] Foster-Powell K, Holt SH, Brand-Miller JC. International table of glycemic index and glycemic load values: 2002.Am J Clin Nutr. 2002 Jul;76(1):5-56.

[59] Parks EJ, Hellerstein MK. Carbohydrate-induced hypertriacylglycerolemia: historical perspective and review of biological mechanisms. *Am J Clin Nutr*. 2000; 71: 412–433.

[60] Liu S, Willett WC, Stampfer MJ, Hu FB, Franz M, Sampson L, Hennekens CH, Manson JE. A prospective study of dietary glycemic load, carbohydrate intake, and risk of coronary heart disease in US women. Am J Clin Nutr. 2000 Jun;71(6):1455-61.

[61] Salmeron J, Ascherio A, Rimm EB, Colditz GA, Spiegelman D, Jenkins DJ, Stampfer MJ, Wing AL, Willett WC. Dietary fiber, glycemic load, and risk of NIDDM in men. Diabetes Care. 1997 Apr;20(4):545-50.

[62] American Diabetes Association, Inc. Evidence-Based Nutrition Principles and Recommendations for the Treatment and Prevention of Diabetes and Related Complications. (Position Statement). Diabetes Care; 25:S50-S60, 2002

[63] National Center for Health Statistics. Vital Statistics of the United States. Available at: http://www.cdc.gov/nchs/products/pubs/pubd/vsus/vsus.htm

[64] Keys A. Atherolsclerosis: A problem in newer public health. Journal of

Mounta Sinai Hospital 10, 118-139, 1953.

[65] Yerushalmy J, Hilleboe HE. Fat in the diet and mortality from heart disease. A methodologic note. New York State Journal of Medicine 1957;57:2343-54.

[66] Ravnskov U. The Cholesterol Myths. Washington: New Trends Publishing, 2000; ISBN 0-9670897-0-0

[67] Yerushalmy J, Hilleboe HE. Fat in the diet and mortality from heart disease. A methodologic note. New York State Journal of Medicine 1957;57:2343-54.

[68] Keys A. Seven countries: a multivariate analysis of death and coronary heart disease. London: Harvard University Press, 1980.

[69] Keys, A. Coronary Heart Disease In Seven Countries. Circulation, 41, suppl. 1, 1-211, 1970.

[70] Anderson KM, Castelli WP, Levy D.   Cholesterol and mortality. 30 years of follow-up from the Framingham study. JAMA. 1987 Apr 24;257(16):2176-80.

[71] Kannell WB. The role of cholesterol in coronary atherogenesis. Medical Clinics of North America 58, 363-379, 1974.

[72] Anderson KM, Castelli WP, Levy D.   Cholesterol and mortality. 30 years of follow-up from the Framingham study. JAMA. 1987 Apr 24;257(16):2176-80.

[73] Castelli, William, Arch Int Med, Jul 1992, 152:7:1371-1372

[74] Gordon T, Kagan A, Garcia-Palmieri M, Kannel WB, Zukel WJ, Tillotson J, Sorlie P, Hjortland M. Diet and its relation to coronary heart disease and death in three populations.Circulation. 1981 Mar;63(3):500-15.

[75] Multiple risk factor intervention trial. Risk factor changes and mortality results. Multiple Risk Factor Intervention Trial Research Group JAMA. 1982;248:1465-1477.

[76] Multiple risk factor intervention trial. Risk factor changes and mortality results. Multiple Risk Factor Intervention Trial Research Group JAMA. 1982;248:1465-1477.

[77] Ravnskov U. The Cholesterol Myths. Washington: New Trends Publishing, 2000; ISBN 0-9670897-0-0.

[78] Mensink RP, Katan MB. Effect of a dietary fatty acids on serum lipids and lipoproteins - A meta-analysis of 27 trials. Arteriosclerosis Thromb 12: 911-919

(1992)

[79] Yu S, Derr J, Etherton T, Kris-Etherton PM. Plasma cholesterol-predictive equations demonstrate that stearic acid is neutral and monounsaturated fatty acids are hypocholesterolemic. Am J Clin Nutr 1995;61:1129-39.

[80] The Lipid Research Clinics Coronary Primary Prevention Trial results. I. Reduction in incidence of coronary heart disease. JAMA. 1984 Jan 20;251(3):351-64.

[81] Kronmal R, Commentary on the published results of the Lipid Research Clinics Coronary Primary Prevention Trial JAMA, April 12, 1985, 253:14:2091

[82] The coronary primary prevention trial: design and implementation: the Lipid Research Clinics Program. J Chronic Dis. 1979;32(9-10):609-31.

[83] The Lipid Research Clinics Coronary Primary Prevention Trial. Results of 6 years of post-trial follow-up. The Lipid Research Clinics Investigators.Arch Intern Med. 1992 Jul;152(7):1399-410.

[84] Howard BV et al. Low-Fat Dietary Pattern and Risk of Cardiovascular Disease. JAMA 2006 Feb 8;295(6):655-666

[85] Beresford S, Low-Fat Dietary Pattern and Risk of Colorectal Cancer: The Women's Health Initiative Randomized Controlled Dietary Modification Trial JAMA. 2006 Feb 8;295:643-654.

[86] Prentice RL, Low-Fat Dietary Pattern and Risk of Invasive Breast Cancer: The Women's Health Initiative Randomized Controlled Dietary Modification Trial. JAMA. 2006 Feb 8;295:629-642.

[87] Parks EJ. Effect of dietary carbohydrate on triglyceride metabolism in humans. J Nutr. 2001 Oct;131(10):2772S-2774S.

[88] Mensink RP, Zock PL, Kester AD, Katan MB. Effects of dietary fatty acids and carbohydrates on the ratio of serum total to HDL cholesterol and on serum lipids and apolipoproteins: a meta-analysis of 60 controlled trials. Am J Clin Nutr. 2003 May;77(5):1146-55.

[89] Ornish, D. Was Dr. Atkins right? J Am Diet Assoc. 2004 Apr;104(4):537-42.

[90] Kassirer JP. Why Should We Swallow What These Studies Say? AEI-Brookings Joint Center Policy Matters 04-22. August 2004. http://www.aei.brook.edu/policy/page.php?id=192&printversion=1 (accessed May 31, 2006)

[91] Huffman, M. USDA Committee Violated Sunshine Law - United States Department of Agriculture - Brief Article Dairy Foods, Nov, 2000 by J. Mark

[92] National Center for Health Statistics. Vital Statistics of the United States. Available at: http://www.cdc.gov/nchs/products/pubs/pubd/vsus/vsus.htm

[93] Nestle, M. Food Politics: How the Food Industry Influences Nutrition and Health. University of California Press. 2002.

[94] CBS News. Citrus Growers Are Steamed. Jan. 22, 2004. http://www.cbsnews.com/stories/2004/01/22/health/main595094.shtml Accessed May 31, 2006.

[95] CBS News Helathwatch. Sugar Lobbyists Sour On Study. London, April 23, 2003. http://www.cbsnews.com/stories/2003/04/23/health/main550727.shtml (accessed May 31, 2006)

[96] Letter from the Department of Health and Human Services to the Director General of the World Health Organization. Available on the Internet at http://www.commercialalert.org/bushadmincomment.pdf

[97] Nestle, M. Fight on Obesity Faces Hefty Commercial Problems. New York Newsday, June 22, 2000

[98] Franz, M.J. et al. Evidence-Based Nutrition Principles and Recommendations for the Treatment and Prevention of Diabetes and Related Complications (Technical Report) Diabetes Care 25:148-198, 2002. http://care.diabetesjournals.org/cgi/content/full/25/1/148. Accessed May 31, 2006.

[99] Trecroci, D. The Biggest Diabetes Busts of All Time. (According to Diabetes Health Readers) Diabetes Health, Jan 2005.

[100] American Diabetes Association. Standards of Medical Care in Diabetes. Diabetes Care 28:S4-S36, 2005

[101] American Diabetes Association. Standards of Medical Care in Diabetes. Diabetes Care 28:S4-S36, 2005

[102] ADA website corporate sponsorship 2003 page: http://www.diabetes.org/aboutus/sponsors/recognize.jsp (accessed January 24, 2004)

[103] St. Joer TS and others. Dietary protein and weight reduction. Circulation 104:1869-1974, 2001.

[104] American Diabetes Association, Inc. Evidence-Based Nutrition Principles and Recommendations for the Treatment and Prevention of Diabetes and Related Complications. (Position Statement). Diabetes Care; 25:S50-S60, 2002

[105] Keys, A. Coronary Heart Disease In Seven Countries. Circulation, 41, suppl. 1, 1-211, 1970.

[106] de Lorgeril M, Salen P, Martin JL, Monjaud I, Delaye J, Mamelle N. Mediterranean diet, traditional risk factors, and the rate of cardiovascular complications after myocardial infarction: final report of the Lyon Diet Heart Study. Circulation. 1999 Feb 16;99(6):779-85.

[107] de Lorgeril M, Salen P, Martin JL, Monjaud I, Delaye J, Mamelle N. Mediterranean diet, traditional risk factors, and the rate of cardiovascular complications after myocardial infarction: final report of the Lyon Diet Heart Study. Circulation. 1999 Feb 16;99(6):779-85.

[108] de Lorgeril M, Salen P, Martin JL, Monjaud I, Boucher P, Mamelle N. Mediterranean dietary pattern in a randomized trial: prolonged survival and possible reduced cancer rate. Arch Intern Med. 1998 Jun 8;158(11):1181-7.

[109] American Heart Association Lyon Diet Heart Study web page. http://www.americanheart.org/presenter.jhtml?identifier=4655 Accessed Oct 26, 2005.

[110] Stephen AM, Wald NJ. Trends in individual consumption of dietary fat in the United States, 1920-1984. Am J of Clin Nutr 1990; 52:457-69

[111] Daily Dietary Fat and Total Food-Energy Intakes-Third National Health and Nutrition Examination Survey, Phase 1, 1988-1991. MMWR 1994; 43:116-117

[112] Alabama Center For Health Statistics. HEART DISEASE DEATHS AND DEATH RATES1 BY RACE AND TOTAL UNITED STATES RATES ALABAMA, 1960-2002 http://ph.state.al.us/chs/HealthStatistics/Tables/2002/AVS02_39.htm

[113] American Heart Association. Heart Disease and Stroke Statistics— 2004 Update. Dallas, Tex.: American Heart Association; 2003.

[114] USDA Center for Nutrition Policy and Promotion. Is total fat consumption really decreasing? Nutrition Insights 5. April 1998

[115] Putnam JJ, Allshouse JE. Food consumption, Prices, and Expenditures, 1970-1997. Washington DC: USDA, 1999.

[116] Putnam JJ, Allshouse JE. Food consumption and Spending, U.S. Per Capita Food Supply Trends. Washington DC: USDA, 1998.
http://www.ers.usda.gov/publications/foodreview/sep1998/frsept98a.pdf

[117] Putnam JJ, Allshouse JE. Food consumption and Spending, U.S. Per Capita Food Supply Trends. Washington DC: USDA, 1998.
http://www.ers.usda.gov/publications/foodreview/sep1998/frsept98a.pdf

[118] Goldstein DJ. Beneficial health effects of modest weight loss. Int J Obes Relat Metab Disord. 1992 Jun;16(6):397-415. Review.

[119] Pan XR, et al. Effects of diet and exercise in preventing NIDDM in people with impaired glucose tolerance. The Da Qing IGT and Diabetes Study. Diabetes Care. 1997 Apr;20(4):537-44.

[120] McCullough ML, Feskanich D, Rimm EB, Giovannucci EL, Ascherio A, Variyam JN, Spiegelman D, Stampfer MJ, Willett WC. Adherence to the Dietary Guidelines for Americans and risk of major chronic disease in men. Am J Clin Nutr. 2000 Nov;72(5):1223-31.

[121] McCullough ML, Feskanich D, Stampfer MJ, Rosner BA, Hu FB, Hunter DJ, Variyam JN, Colditz GA, Willett WC. Adherence to the Dietary Guidelines for Americans and risk of major chronic disease in women. Am J Clin Nutr. 2000 Nov;72(5):1214-22.

[122] Taubes G. Nutrition. The soft science of dietary fat. Science. 2001 Mar 30;291(5513):2536-45.

[123] Beresford S, Low-Fat Dietary Pattern and Risk of Colorectal Cancer: The Women's Health Initiative Randomized Controlled Dietary Modification Trial JAMA. 2006 Feb 8;295:643-654.

[124] Hu FB, Stampfer MJ, Manson JE, Rimm E, Colditz GA, Rosner BA, Hennekens CH, Willett WC. Dietary fat intake and the risk of coronary heart disease in women. N Engl J Med. 1997 Nov 20;337(21):1491-9.

[125] Willett WC. Dietary fat plays a major role in obesity: no. Obes Rev. 2002 May;3(2):59-68.

[126] Willett WC, Leibel RL. Dietary fat is not a major determinant of body fat. Am J Med. 2002 Dec 30;113 Suppl 9B:47S-59S.

[127] Willett WC. Dietary fat plays a major role in obesity: no. Obes Rev. 2002 May;3(2):59-68.

[128] Harper CR, Jacobson TA.   Beyond the Mediterranean diet: the role of omega-3 Fatty acids in the prevention of coronary heart disease. Prev Cardiol. 2003 Summer;6(3):136-46.

[129] Covington MB. Omega-3 fatty acids. Am Fam Physician. 2004 Jul 1;70(1):133-40. Review.

[130] Dietary supplementation with n-3 polyunsaturated fatty acids and vitamin E after myocardial infarction: results of the GISSI-Prevenzione trial. Gruppo Italiano per lo Studio della Sopravvivenza nell'Infarto miocardico. Lancet. 1999; 354: 447–455.

[131] Singh RB, Niaz MA, Sharma JP, et al. Randomized, double-blind, placebo-controlled trial of fish oil and mustard oil in patients with suspected acute myocardial infarction: the Indian experiment of infarct survival-4. Cardiovasc Drugs Ther. 1997; 11: 485–491.

[132] Burr ML, Fehily AM, Gilbert JF, et al. Effects of changes in fat, fish, and fibre intakes on death and myocardial reinfarction: diet and reinfarction trial (DART). Lancet. 1989; 2: 757–761

[133] Bucher HC, Hengstler P, Schindler C, et al. N-3 polyunsaturated fatty acids in coronary heart disease: a meta-analysis of randomized controlled trials. Am J Med. 2002; 112: 298–304.

[134] de Lorgeril M, Salen P, Martin JL, Monjaud I, Delaye J, Mamelle N. Mediterranean diet, traditional risk factors, and the rate of cardiovascular complications after myocardial infarction: final report of the Lyon Diet Heart Study. Circulation. 1999 Feb 16;99(6):779-85.

[135] Mensink RP, Katan MB.Effect of dietary fatty acids on serum lipids and lipoproteins. A meta-analysis of 27 trials. Arterioscler Thromb. 1992 Aug;12(8):911-9.

[136] Hu FB, Stampfer MJ, Manson JE, Rimm E, Colditz GA, Rosner BA, Hennekens CH, Willett WC. Dietary fat intake and the risk of coronary heart disease in women.

[137] Salmeron J, Hu FB, Manson JE, Stampfer MJ, Colditz GA, Rimm EB, Willett WC. Dietary fat intake and risk of type 2 diabetes in women. Am J Clin Nutr. 2001 Jun;73(6):1019-26.

[138] Katan MB, Zock PL, Mensink RP. Effects of fats and fatty acids on blood lipids in humans: an overview. Am J Clin Nutr. 1994 Dec;60(6 Suppl):1017S-

1022S. Review.

[139] Low, CC. Potentiation of the effects of weight loss by monounsaturated fatty acids in obese NIDDM patients.

[140] McManus K, Antinoro L, Sacks F. A randomized controlled trial of a moderate-fat, low-energy diet compared with a low fat, low-energy diet for weight loss in overweight adults. Int J Obes Relat Metab Disord. 2001 Oct;25(10):1503-11.

[141] Yu S, Derr J, Etherton T, Kris-Etherton PM. Plasma cholesterol-predictive equations demonstrate that stearic acid is neutral and monounsaturated fatty acids are hypocholesterolemic. Am J Clin Nutr 1995;61:1129-39.

[142] Oh K, Hu FB, Manson JE, Stampfer MJ, Willett WC. Dietary fat intake and risk of coronary heart disease in women: 20 years of follow-up of the nurses' health study. Am J Epidemiol. 2005 Apr 1;161(7):672-9.

[143] Ascherio A, Rimm EB, Giovannucci EL, Spiegelman D, Stampfer M, Willett WC. Dietary fat and risk of coronary heart disease in men: cohort follow up study in the United States.BMJ. 1996 Jul 13;313(7049):84-90.

[144] Zock PL, Mensink RP. Dietary trans-fatty acids and serum lipoproteins in humans.Curr Opin Lipidol. 1996 Feb;7(1):34-7.

[145] Hu FB, Stampfer MJ, Manson JE, Rimm E, Colditz GA, Rosner BA, Hennekens CH, Willett WC. Dietary fat intake and the risk of coronary heart disease in women.

[146] Salmeron J, Hu FB, Manson JE, Stampfer MJ, Colditz GA, Rimm EB, Willett WC. Dietary fat intake and risk of type 2 diabetes in women. Am J Clin Nutr. 2001 Jun;73(6):1019-26.

[147] Enig, Mary G, PhD, Trans Fatty Acids in the Food Supply: A Comprehensive Report Covering 60 Years of Research, 2nd Edition, Enig Associates, Inc, Silver Spring, MD, 1995; Watkins, B A et al, Br Pouli Sci, Dec 1991, 32(5):1109-1119

[148] Enig, "Know Your Fats: The Complete Primer for Understanding the Nutrition of Fats, Oils and Cholesterol", Bethesda Press, 14 May, 2000.

[149] Anderson JW. Dietary fiber prevents carbohydrate-induced hypertriglyceridemia. Curr Atheroscler Rep. 2000 Nov;2(6):536-41. Review.

[150] Chandalia M, Garg A, Lutjohann D, von Bergmann K, Grundy SM, Brinkley LJ. Beneficial effects of high dietary fiber intake in patients with type 2 diabetes

mellitus.

N Engl J Med. 2000 May 11;342(19):1392-8.

[151] Salmeron J, Hu FB, Manson JE, Stampfer MJ, Colditz GA, Rimm EB, Willett WC. Dietary fat intake and risk of type 2 diabetes in women. Am J Clin Nutr. 2001 Jun;73(6):1019-26.

[152] Salmeron J, Ascherio A, Rimm EB, Colditz GA, Spiegelman D, Jenkins DJ, Stampfer MJ, Wing AL, Willett WC. Dietary fiber, glycemic load, and risk of NIDDM in men. Diabetes Care. 1997 Apr;20(4):545-50.

[153] Pereira MA, O'Reilly E, Augustsson K, Fraser GE, Goldbourt U, Heitmann BL, Hallmans G, Knekt P, Liu S, Pietinen P, Spiegelman D, Stevens J, Virtamo J, Willett WC, Ascherio A. Dietary fiber and risk of coronary heart disease: a pooled analysis of cohort studies. Arch Intern Med. 2004 Feb 23;164(4):370-6.

[154] Brand Miller, J. et al, The new glucose revolution pocket guide to diabetes. Rev. and expanded ed. 2003, New York: Marlowe & Co. University of Sydney online Glycemic Index Database http://www.glycemicindex.com/

[155] Brand Miller, J. et al, The new glucose revolution pocket guide to diabetes. Rev. and expanded ed. 2003, New York: Marlowe & Co. University of Sydney online Glycemic Index Database http://www.glycemicindex.com/

[156] Wolever TM. Relationship between dietary fiber content and composition in foods and the glycemic index. Am J Clin Nutr. 1990 Jan;51(1):72-5.

[157] Brand Miller, J. et al, The new glucose revolution pocket guide to diabetes. Rev. and expanded ed. 2003, New York: Marlowe & Co. University of Sydney online Glycemic Index Database http://www.glycemicindex.com/

[158] Brand Miller, J. et al, The new glucose revolution pocket guide to diabetes. Rev. and expanded ed. 2003, New York: Marlowe & Co. University of Sydney online Glycemic Index Database http://www.glycemicindex.com/

[159] Gilbertson HR, Brand-Miller JC, Thorburn AW, Evans S, Chondros P, Werther GA. The effect of flexible low glycemic index dietary advice versus measured carbohydrate exchange diets on glycemic control in children with type 1 diabetes. Diabetes Care. 2001 Jul;24(7):1137-43.

[160] American Dietetic Association. Fat replacers. Position statement. http://www.eatright.org/Public/Other/index_adap0498.cfm

[161] Cotton JR, Weststrate JA, Blundell JE. Replacement of dietary fat with

sucrose polyester: effects on energy intake and appetite control in nonobese males. Am J Clin Nutr. 1996 Jun;63(6):891-6.

[162] Stubbs RJ.   The effect of ingesting olestra-based foods on feeding behavior and energy balance in humans. Crit Rev Food Sci Nutr. 2001 Jul;41(5):363-86. Review. PMID: 11497329

[163] Wright JD, Kennedy-Stephenson J, Wang CY, McDowell MA, Johnson CL. Trends in intake of energy and macronutrients-united states, 1971-2000 Mor Mortal Wkly Rep 2004;6:80-82. http://www.cdc.gov/mmwr/preview/mmwrhtml/mm5304a3.htm.

[164] Centers for Disease Control and Prevention. Monitoring the Nation's Health. Dietary intake of macronutrients, micronutrients, and other dietary constituents: United states, 1988-1994 Vital Health Stat 2002;11:9-85.

[165] Mensink RP, Zock PL, Kester AD, Katan MB. Effects of dietary fatty acids and carbohydrates on the ratio of serum total to HDL cholesterol and on serum lipids and apolipoproteins: a meta-analysis of 60 controlled trials. Am J Clin Nutr. 2003 May;77(5):1146-55.

[166] Salmeron J, Hu FB, Manson JE, Stampfer MJ, Colditz GA, Rimm EB, Willett WC. Dietary fat intake and risk of type 2 diabetes in women. Am J Clin Nutr. 2001 Jun;73(6):1019-26.

[167] Oh K, Hu FB, Manson JE, Stampfer MJ, Willett WC. Dietary Fat Intake and Risk of Coronary Heart Disease in Women: 20 Years of Follow-up of the Nurses' Health Study. Am J Epidemiol. 2005 Apr 1;161(7):672-9. PMID: 15781956 [PubMed - in process]

[168] Mozaffarian D, Ascherio A, Hu FB, Stampfer MJ, Willett WC, Siscovick DS, Rimm EB. Interplay between different polyunsaturated fatty acids and risk of coronary heart disease in men. Circulation. 2005 Jan 18;111(2):157-64. Epub 2005 Jan 3.

[169] Iso H, Rexrode KM, Stampfer MJ, Manson JE, Colditz GA, Speizer FE, Hennekens CH, Willett WC. Intake of fish and omega-3 fatty acids and risk of stroke in women. JAMA. 2001 Jan 17;285(3):304-12.

[170] Mensink RP, Zock PL, Kester AD, Katan MB. Effects of dietary fatty acids and carbohydrates on the ratio of serum total to HDL cholesterol and on serum lipids and apolipoproteins: a meta-analysis of 60 controlled trials. Am J Clin Nutr. 2003 May;77(5):1146-55.

[171] Aspartame Victims Support Group. Ninety-two symptoms reported to the
FDA in 1995, on US Department of Health and Human Services stationary,
obtained with the freedom of information act.
http://www.presidiotex.com/aspartame/Facts/92_Symptoms/92_symptoms.html

[172] Walton RG, Survey of aspartame studies: correlation of outcome and funding
sources http://www.presidiotex.com/aspartame/index.html

[173] Cohen J, THE EFFECTS OF DIFFERENT STORAGE TEMPERATURES
ON THE TASTE AND CHEMICAL COMPOSITION OF DIET COKE, Food
Chemical News, 5 May, 1997 (Volume 39 No.11)

[174] http://www.stevia.net/fda.htm

[175] http://www.stevia.net/bookburning.htm

[176] Natah SS, Hussien KR, Tuominen JA, Koivisto VA: Metabolic response to
lactitol and xylitol in healthy men. Am J Clin Nutr 65:947–950, 1997

[177] Wheeler ML, Fineberg SE, Gibson R, Fineberg N: Metabolic response to oral
challenge of hydrogenated starch hydrolysates versus glucose in diabetes.
Diabetes Care 13:733–740, 1990

[178] Akgun S, Ertel NH: A comparison of carbohydrate metabolism after sucrose,
sorbitol, and fructose meals in normal and diabetic subjects. Diabetes Care
3:582–585, 1980

[179] Rizkalla SW, Luo J, Wils D, Bruzzo F, Slama G. Glycaemic and insulinaemic
responses to a new hydrogenated starch hydrolysate in healthy and type 2
diabetic subjects. Diabetes Metab. 2002 Nov;28(5):385-90.

[180] Livesey G: Health potential of polyols as sugar replacers, with emphasis on
low glycaemic properties. Nutrition Research Reviews, December 2003, vol. 16,
no. 2, pp. 163-191(29)

[181] Vernia P, Frandina C, Bolotta T, Ricciardi MR, Vollotti G, Fallucca F:
Sorbitol malabsorption and nonspecific abdominal symptoms in type II diabetes.
Metabolism 44:796–799, 1995

[182] Payne ML, Craig WJ, Williams AC: Sorbitol is a possible risk factor for
diarrhea in young children. J Am Diet Assoc 97:532–534, 1997

[183] Jain NK, Rosenberg DB, Ulahannan MJ, Glasser MJ, Pitchumoni CS:
Sorbitol intolerance in adults. J Gastroenterol 80:678–681, 1985

[184] Zock PL, Mensink RP. Dietary trans-fatty acids and serum lipoproteins in

humans.Curr Opin Lipidol. 1996 Feb;7(1):34-7.

[185] Hu FB, Stampfer MJ, Manson JE, Rimm E, Colditz GA, Rosner BA, Hennekens CH, Willett WC. Dietary fat intake and the risk of coronary heart disease in women.

[186] Salmeron J, Hu FB, Manson JE, Stampfer MJ, Colditz GA, Rimm EB, Willett WC. Dietary fat intake and risk of type 2 diabetes in women. Am J Clin Nutr. 2001 Jun;73(6):1019-26.

[187] Enig, Mary G, PhD, Trans Fatty Acids in the Food Supply: A Comprehensive Report Covering 60 Years of Research, 2nd Edition, Enig Associates, Inc, Silver Spring, MD, 1995; Watkins, B A et al, Br Pouli Sci, Dec 1991, 32(5):1109-1119

[188] Final Report: Assessment of the Dose-Response Effect of Olestra on the Status of Fat-Soluble Vitamins and Other Marker Nutrients in Humans. Submitted by P&G to the FDA on January 29, 1993.

[189] Weststrate JA, van het Hof KH. Sucrose polyester and plasma carotenoid concentrations in healthy subjects. Am J Clin Nutr. 1995 Sep;62(3):591-7. PMID: 7661121

[190] New Actions Opposing Olestra. CSPI Press release. June 10, 1998 http://www.cspinet.org/new/oles_6_9.htm

[191] Michigan Today. Fall 1996. http://www.umich.edu/~newsinfo/MT/96/Fall96/mta1f96.html

[192] J Lazarou, BM Pomeranz, PN Corey. Incidence of Adverse Drug Reactions in hospitalized patients: A Meta-Analysis of prospective studies. JAMA 1998 279: 1200-5.

[193] Crosse, M. Dietary Supplements Containing Ephedra Health Risks and FDA's Oversight. Testimony Before the Subcommittee on Oversight and Investigations, Committee on Energy and Commerce, House of Representatives. July 23, 2003. http://www.gao.gov/new.items/d031042t.pdf

[194] Bendich A, Mallick R, Leader S. Potential health economic benefits of vitamin supplementation. Western J Medicine 1997;166:306-312.

[195] CBSNews.com consumer report Get-Rich-Quick Plan A Scam? June 4, 2004 http://www.cbsnews.com/stories/2004/06/04/eveningnews/consumer/main62121 3.shtml Accessed July 18, 2006

[196] Barrett, S and Herbert, V. The Vitamin Pushers, How the "Health Food"

Industry Is Selling America a Bill of Goods. Prometheus Books, New York, 1994.

[197] Lewis C. Investigators' Reports Dietary Supplement Maker Fined Twice What Company Profited http://www.fda.gov/Fdac/departs/2001/101_irs.html

[198] Taylor, J. United States Senate Special Committee on Aging Hearing on Swindlers, Hucksters and Snake Oil Salesmen: The Hype and Hope of Marketing Anti-Aging Products to Seniors. September 10, 2001

http://www.quackwatch.org/01QuackeryRelatedTopics/Hearing/taylor.html

[199] Crosse, M. Dietary Supplements Containing Ephedra Health Risks and FDA's Oversight. Testimony Before the Subcommittee on Oversight and Investigations, Committee on Energy and Commerce, House of Representatives. July 23, 2003. http://www.gao.gov/new.items/d031042t.pdf

[200] Barrett, S and Herbert, V. The Vitamin Pushers, How the "Health Food" Industry Is Selling America a Bill of Goods. Prometheus Books, New York, 1994.

[201] Barrett, S and Herbert, V. The Vitamin Pushers, How the "Health Food" Industry Is Selling America a Bill of Goods. Prometheus Books, New York, 1994.

[202] http://groups.google.com/group/alt.support.diabetes/browse_frm/thread/cec4af a4446e9838/a3805abb131c4f62? Accessed, May 31, 2006.

[203] http://naturalcurves.tripod.com/naturalcurves_sp825.html Accessed, May 31, 2006.

[204] Web site: http://www.advancedhealthgroup.com/nutrition_nutrition.html

[205] Nutrition 21 Marketing Literature. http://www.nutrition21.com/About/default.aspx. Accesed May 31, 2006.

[206] Nutrition 21 Marketing Literature. http://www.nutrition21.com/About/default.aspx Accessed May 31, 2006.

[207] Althuis MD, Jordan NE, Ludington EA, Wittes JT. Glucose and insulin responses to dietary chromium supplements: a meta-analysis. Am J Clin Nutr. 2002 Jul;76(1):148-55.

[208] Speetjens JK, Collins RA, Vincent JB, Woski SA. The nutritional supplement chromium(III) tris(picolinate) cleaves DNA. Chem Res Toxicol. 1999 Jun;12(6):483-7.

[209] Anderson RA, Cheng N, Bryden NA, Polansky MM, Cheng N, Chi J, Feng J. Elevated intakes of supplemental chromium improve glucose and insulin variables in individuals with type 2 diabetes. Diabetes. 1997 Nov;46(11):1786-91.

[210] Bahijiri SM, Mira SA, Mufti AM, Ajabnoor MA. The effects of inorganic chromium and brewer's yeast supplementation on glucose tolerance, serum lipids and drug dosage in individuals with type 2 diabetes. Saudi Med J. 2000 Sep;21(9):831-7.

[211] Anderson RA, Roussel AM, Zouari N, Mahjoub S, Matheau JM, Kerkeni A. Potential antioxidant effects of zinc and chromium supplementation in people with type 2 diabetes mellitus. J Am Coll Nutr. 2001 Jun;20(3):212-8.

[212] Thomas VL, Gropper SS. Effect of chromium nicotinic acid supplementation on selected cardiovascular disease risk factors. Biol Trace Elem Res. 1996 Dec;55(3):297-305.

[213] Lee NA, Reasner CA. Beneficial effect of chromium supplementation on serum triglyceride levels in NIDDM. Diabetes Care. 1994 Dec;17(12):1449-52.

[214] Abraham AS, Brooks BA, Eylath U. The effects of chromium supplementation on serum glucose and lipids in patients with and without non-insulin-dependent diabetes. Metabolism. 1992 Jul;41(7):768-71.

[215] Barrett, S and Herbert, V. The Vitamin Pushers, How the "Health Food" Industry Is Selling America a Bill of Goods. Prometheus Books, New York, 1994. (pp 87-89, 154-155)

[216] Maxwell SRJ, Thomason H, Sandler D, Leguen C, Baxter MA, Thorpe GHG, Jones AF, Barnett AH 1997 Antioxidant status in patients with uncomplicated insulin-dependent and non-insulin-dependent diabetes mellitus. Eur J Clin Invest 27:484–490

[217] Hartnett ME, Stratton RD, Browne RW, Rosner BA, Lanham RJ, Armstrong D 2000 Serum markers for oxidative stress and severity of diabetic retinopathy. Diabetes Care 23:234–240

[218] Salonen JT, Nyyssonen K, Tuomainen TP, Maenpaa PH, Korpela H, Kaplan GA, Lynch J, Helmrich SP, Salonen R 1995 Increased risk of non-insulin dependent diabetes mellitus at low plasma vitamin E concentrations: a four year follow up study in men. BMJ 311:1124–1127

[219] Opara EC, Abdel-Rahman E, Soliman S, Kamel WA, Souka S, Lowe JE,

Abdel-Aleem S 1999 Depletion of total antioxidant capacity in type 2 diabetes. Metabolism 48:1414–1417

[220] Vanroelen WF, Van Gaal LF, Van Rooy PE, De Leeuw IH. Serum and erythrocyte magnesium levels in type I & type II diabetics. Acta Diabetol Lat 1985;22:185–90.

[221] Mooradian AD, Morley JE. Micronutrient status in diabetes mellitus. Am J Clin Nutr 1987;45:877–95.

[222] Smith RG, Heise CC, King JC, Costa FM, Kitzmiller JL. Serum and urinary magnesium, calcium and copper levels in insulin dependent diabetic women. J Trace Elem Electrolytes Health Dis 1988;2:239–43.

[223] Paolisso G, Scheen A, D'Onofrio FD, Lefebvre P. Magnesium and glucose homeostasis. Diabetologia 1990;33:511–4

[224] Cunningham JJ, Ellis SL, McVeigh KL, et al. Reduced mononuclear leukocyte ascorbic acid content in adults with insulin-dependent diabetes mellitus consuming adequate dietary vitamin C. Metabolism 1991;40:146–9.

[225] Wilson RG, Davis RE. Serum pyridoxal concentrations in children with diabetes mellitus. Pathology 1977;9:95–9.

[226] Davis RE, Calder JS, Curnow DH. Serum pyridoxal and folate concentrations in diabetics. Pathology 1976;8:151–6.

[227] Nakamura T, Higashi A, Nishiyama S, et al. Kinetics of zinc status in children with IDDM. Diabetes Care 1991;14:553–7.

[228] Holt SH, Miller JC, Petocz P, Farmakalidis E. A satiety index of common foods. Eur J Clin Nutr. 1995 Sep;49(9):675-90.

[229] Diabetes Prevention Research Group: Reduction in the evidence of type 2 diabetes with life-style intervention or metformin. New England Journal of Medicine 346:393-403, 2002.

[230] Lindstrom J, Louheranta A, Mannelin M, Rastas M, Salminen V, Eriksson J, Uusitupa M, Tuomilehto J; Finnish Diabetes Prevention Study Group. The Finnish Diabetes Prevention Study (DPS): Lifestyle intervention and 3-year results on diet and physical activity. Diabetes Care. 2003 Dec;26(12):3230-6.

[231] Pan XR, Li GW, Hu YH, Wang JX, Yang WY, An ZX, Hu ZX, Lin J, Xiao JZ, Cao HB, Liu PA, Jiang XG, Jiang YY, Wang JP, Zheng H, Zhang H, Bennett PH, Howard BV. Effects of diet and exercise in preventing NIDDM in

people with impaired glucose tolerance. The Da Qing IGT and Diabetes Study. Diabetes Care. 1997 Apr;20(4):537-44.

[232] Diabetes Control and Complications Trial Research Group: The effect of intensive treatment of diabetes on the development and progression of long-term complications in insulin-dependent diabetes mellitus. N Engl J Med 329:977–986, 1993

[233] Reichard P, Nilsson BY, Rosenqvist V: The effect of long-term intensified insulin treatment on the development of microvascular complications of diabetes mellitus. N Engl J Med 329:304–309, 1993

[234] University Group Diabetes Program. A study of the effects of hypoglycemic agents on vascular complications in patients with adult-onset diabetes. Diabetes 1970; 19 (suppl 2): 747–830.

[235] University Group Diabetes Program.A study of the effects of hypoglycemic agents on vascular complications in patients with adult-onset diabetes. V. Evaluation of phenformin therapy. Diabetes 1975; 24 (suppl 1): 65–184.

[236] Seltzer HS. A summary of criticisms of the findings and conclusions of the University Group Diabetes Program (UGDP). Diabetes 1972; 21(9):976-9.

[237] Intensive blood-glucose control with sulphonylureas or insulin compared with conventional treatment and risk of complications in patients with type 2 diabetes (UKPDS 33). UK Prospective Diabetes Study (UKPDS) Group. Lancet. 1998 Sep 12;352(9131):837-53.

[238] Intensive blood-glucose control with sulphonylureas or insulin compared with conventional treatment and risk of complications in patients with type 2 diabetes (UKPDS 33). UK Prospective Diabetes Study (UKPDS) Group. Lancet. 1998 Sep 12;352(9131):837-53.

[239] Intensive blood-glucose control with sulphonylureas or insulin compared with conventional treatment and risk of complications in patients with type 2 diabetes (UKPDS 33). UK Prospective Diabetes Study (UKPDS) Group. Lancet. 1998 Sep 12;352(9131):837-53.

[240] Intensive blood-glucose control with sulphonylureas or insulin compared with conventional treatment and risk of complications in patients with type 2 diabetes (UKPDS 33). UK Prospective Diabetes Study (UKPDS) Group. Lancet. 1998 Sep 12;352(9131):837-53.

[241] American Diabetes Association. Implications of the United Kingdom

Prospective Diabetes Study Diabetes Care 25:S28-S32, 2002

[242] Intensive blood-glucose control with sulphonylureas or insulin compared with conventional treatment and risk of complications in patients with type 2 diabetes (UKPDS 33). UK Prospective Diabetes Study (UKPDS) Group. Lancet. 1998 Sep 12;352(9131):837-53.

[243] Stratton IM, Adler AI, Neil HA, Matthews DR, Manley SE, Cull CA, Hadden D, Turner RC, Holman RR. Association of glycaemia with macrovascular and microvascular complications of type 2 diabetes (UKPDS 35): prospective observational study. BMJ. 2000 Aug 12;321(7258):405-12.

[244] Effect of intensive blood-glucose control with metformin on complications in overweight patients with type 2 diabetes (UKPDS 34). UK Prospective Diabetes Study (UKPDS) Group.
Lancet. 1998 Sep 12;352(9131):854-65.

[245] Chiquette E, Ramirez G, Defronzo R.   A meta-analysis comparing the effect of thiazolidinediones on cardiovascular risk factors. Arch Intern Med. 2004 Oct 25;164(19):2097-104.

[246] Dailey GE 3rd, Noor MA, Park JS, Bruce S, Fiedorek FT. Glycemic control with glyburide/metformin tablets in combination with rosiglitazone in patients with type 2 diabetes: a randomized, double-blind trial. Am J Med. 2004 Feb 15;116(4):223-9.

[247] Tan M, Johns D, Gonzalez Galvez G, Antunez O, Fabian G, Flores-Lozano F, Zuniga Guajardo S, Garza E, Morales H, Konkoy C, Herz M; GLAD Study Group. Effects of pioglitazone and glimepiride on glycemic control and insulin sensitivity in Mexican patients with type 2 diabetes mellitus: A multicenter, randomized, double-blind, parallel-group trial. Clin Ther. 2004 May;26(5):680-93.

[248] Derosa G, Cicero AF, Gaddi A, Ragonesi PD, Fogari E, Bertone G, Ciccarelli L, Piccinni MN. Metabolic effects of pioglitazone and rosiglitazone in patients with diabetes and metabolic syndrome treated with glimepiride: a twelve-month, multicenter, double-blind, randomized, controlled, parallel-group trial.

[249] Charbonnel BH, Matthews DR, Schernthaner G, Hanefeld M, Brunetti P; QUARTET Study Group. A long-term comparison of pioglitazone and gliclazide in patients with Type 2 diabetes mellitus: a randomized, double-blind, parallel-group comparison trial. Diabet Med. 2005 Apr;22(4):399-405.

[250] Schernthaner G, Matthews DR, Charbonnel B, Hanefeld M, Brunetti P; Quartet [corrected] Study Group. Efficacy and safety of pioglitazone versus metformin in patients with type 2 diabetes mellitus: a double-blind, randomized trial. J Clin Endocrinol Metab. 2004 Dec;89(12):6068-76. Erratum in: J Clin Endocrinol Metab. 2005 Feb;90(2):746.

[251] Rajagopalan R, Iyer S, Khan M. Effect of pioglitazone on metabolic syndrome risk factors: results of double-blind, multicenter, randomized clinical trials. Curr Med Res Opin. 2005 Jan;21(1):163-72.

[252] Olansky L, Marchetti A, Lau H. Multicenter retrospective assessment of thiazolidinedione monotherapy and combination therapy in patients with type 2 diabetes: comparative subgroup analyses of glycemic control and blood lipid levels. Clin Ther. 2003;25 Suppl B:B64-80. Review.

[253] Aljabri K, Kozak SE, Thompson DM. Addition of pioglitazone or bedtime insulin to maximal doses of sulfonylurea and metformin in type 2 diabetes patients with poor glucose control: a prospective, randomized trial. Am J Med. 2004 Feb 15;116(4):230-5.

[254] Haffner SM, Greenberg AS, Weston WM, Chen H, Williams K, Freed MI. Effect of rosiglitazone treatment on nontraditional markers of cardiovascular disease in patients with type 2 diabetes mellitus. Circulation. 2002 Aug 6;106(6):679-84.

[255] Lester JW, Fernandes AW. Pioglitazone in a subgroup of patients with type 2 diabetes meeting the criteria for metabolic syndrome. Int J Clin Pract. 2005 Feb;59(2):134-42.

[256] Intensive blood-glucose control with sulphonylureas or insulin compared with conventional treatment and risk of complications in patients with type 2 diabetes (UKPDS 33). UK Prospective Diabetes Study (UKPDS) Group. Lancet. 1998 Sep 12;352(9131):837-53.

[257] Charbonnel B, Dormandy J, Erdmann E, Massi-Benedetti M, Skene A, on behalf of the PROactive Study Group. The Prospective Pioglitazone Clinical Trial in Macrovascular Events (PROactive). Can pioglitazone reduce cardiovascular events in diabetes? Study design and baseline characteristics of 5238 patients. Diabetes Care 2004;27:1647-53

[258] Home PD, Pocock SJ, Beck-Nielsen H, Gomis R, Hanefeld M, Dargie H, Komajda M, Gubb J, Biswas N, Jones NP. Rosiglitazone Evaluated for Cardiac

Outcomes and Regulation of Glycaemia in Diabetes (RECORD): study design and protocol. Diabetologia. 2005 Jul 16;

[259] Gerstein HC,Rationale, design and recruitment characteristics of a large, simple international trial of diabetes prevention: the DREAM trial.

[260] Starfield, Is US Health Really the Best in the World? Journal of the American Medical Association, July 26, 2000, Vol 284, No 4.

[261] Johnson JA, Bootman JL. Drug-related morbidity and mortality and the economic impact of pharmaceutical care. Am J Health Syst Pharm 1997; 54: 554-558

[262] Ernst FR, Grizzle AJ. Drug-related morbidity and mortality: updating the cost-of-illness model. J Am Pharm Assoc (Wash). 2001 Mar-Apr;41(2):192-9.

[263] Alliance for Aging Research. When Medicine Hurts Instead of Helps. Washington, DC: The Alliance for Aging Research; 1998.

[264] National Institute for Healthcare Management. Prescription Drug Expenditures in 2001: Another Year of Escalating Costs, NIHCM Foundation, March 29, 2002, http://www.nihcm.org/spending2001.pdf

[265] Pfizer Inc., 2004 Financial Report. http://www.pfizer.com/pfizer/are/investors_reports/index.jsp

[266] IMS Health. Press release. March 9, 2005. http://www.imshealth.com/ims/portal/front/articleC/0,2777,6599_3665_714964 63,00.html

[267] The Fortune 500, Fortune Vol. 147, No. 7, April 17, 2003

[268] Angell M., The Truth About Drug Companies: How They Deceive Us and What To Do About It. Random House, New York, 2004.

[269] National Institute For Healthcare Management, Prescription Drugs and Mass Media Advertising, 2000, NIHCM Foundation, November 21, 2001

[270] Pharmacy: Looking Ahead. U.S. Pharm. 2004;8:72. Vol. No: 29:08 http://www.uspharmacist.com/index.asp?show=article&page=8_1322.htm

[271] U.S. Food and Drug Administration "The Pink Sheet: The News This Week" February 19, 2001. From Public Citizen's Congress Watch. America's other drug problem A briefing book on the rx drug debate. http://www.citizen.org/rxfacts

[272] United States of America, ex rel. David Franklin v. Pfizer Inc., and Parke-

Davis, Division of Warner-Lambert Company. Civil Action No. 96-11651 —
PBS. United States District Court for the District of Massachusetts.

[273] Backonja M, Beydoun A, Edwards KR, Schwartz SL, Fonseca V, Hes M,
LaMoreaux L, Garofalo E. Gabapentin for the symptomatic treatment of painful
neuropathy in patients with diabetes mellitus: a randomized controlled trial.
JAMA. 1998 Dec 2;280(21):1831-6.

[274] Schiebel NE, Ebbert J, Margolis K, Backonja M. Gabapentin for painful
diabetic neuropathy. JAMA. 1999 Jul 14;282(2):133-134.

[275]Kaiser family foundation Prescription drug trends.
http://www.kff.org/rxdrugs/market.cfm?

[276] Chin T. "Drug firms score by paying doctors for time," American Medical
News, May 6, 2002.

[277] United States General Accounting Office. "Prescription Drugs: FDA
Oversight of Direct-to-Consumer Advertising Has Limitations" GAO-03-177.
October 2002.

[278] Moynihan R. Who pays for the pizza? Redefining the relationships between
doctors and drug companies. 1: Entanglement BMJ 2003;326:1189-1192 (31
May)

[279] Watkins C, Moore L, Harvey I, Carthy P, Robinson E, Brawn R.
Characteristics of general practitioners who frequently see drug industry
representatives: national cross sectional survey. *BMJ* 2003;326: 1178-9

[280] Wazana A. Physicians and the pharmaceutical industry: is a gift ever just a
gift? JAMA. 2000 Jan 19; 283(3): 373-80.

[281] Katz D, Caplan A, Merz J. All gifts large and small: toward and
understanding of the ethics of pharmaceutical industry gift giving. *Am J
Bioethics* 2003

[282] Hensley S. Health: New Rules Will Push Drug Firms To New Tactics in
Wooing Doctors. The Wall Street Journal. April 23, 2002

[283] Chin, "Drug Firms Score By Paying Doctors For Time"

[284] Moynihan R. Drug company sponsorship of education could be replaced at a
fraction of its cost. BMJ 2003;326:1163 (31 May, 2003).

[285] Relman AS, Angell M. America's other drug problem: how the drug industry
distorts medicine and politics. New Repub. 2002 Dec 16;227(25):27-41.

[286] Jackson, T. Are You Being Duped? How Drug Companies Use Opinion Leaders. BMJ 2003;322:1312.

[287] PBS Science and Health "Now with Bill Moyers" Transcript. Nov 22, 2002. http://www.pbs.org/now/transcript/transcript_scienceforsale.html

[288] Angell M., The Truth About Drug Companies: How They Deceive Us and What To Do About It. p 117. Random House, New York, 2004.

[289] PBS Science and Health "Now with Bill Moyers" Transcript. Nov 22, 2002. http://www.pbs.org/now/transcript/transcript_scienceforsale.html

[290] Joel Lexchin, J, Bero, L, Djulbegovic, B, Clark, O. Pharmaceutical industry sponsorship and research outcome and quality: systematic review. BMJ 2003;326:1167-1170.

[291] Als-Nielsen B, Chen, W, Gluud, C, Kjaergard L. Association of Funding and Conclusions in Randomized Drug TrialsA Reflection of Treatment Effect or Adverse Events? JAMA. 2003;290:921-928.

[292] Bero LA, Rennie D. Influences on the quality of published drug studies. International Journal of Technology Assessment in Health Care 1996;12:209-237.

[293] Bodenheimer T. Uneasy alliance--clinical investigators and the pharmaceutical industry. N Engl J Med. 2000 May 18;342(20):1539-44.

[294] U.S. Food and Drug Administration. Bextra Label Updated with Boxed Warning Concerning Severe Skin Reactions and Warning Regarding Cardiovascular Risk. T04-56. December 9, 2004

[295] United States of America, ex rel. David Franklin v. Pfizer Inc., and Parke-Davis, Division of Warner-Lambert Company. Civil Action No. 96-11651 — PBS. United States District Court for the District of Massachusetts.

[296] Petersen M. In U.S., Madison Ave. Plays Growing Role in Drug Research. The New York Times. Saturday, November 23, 2002

[297] Rochon PA, Berger PB, Gordon M. The evolution of clinical trials: inclusion and representation. CMAJ 1998;159:1373-4.

[298] Rochon PA, Gurwitz JH, Simms RW et al. A study of manufacturer-supported trials of nonsteroidal anti-inflammatory drugs in the treatment of arthritis. Arch Intern Med 1994;154:157-163.

[299] Public Citizen. The Other Drug War: Big Pharma's 625 Washington

Lobbyists. July 2001.
http://www.citizen.org/congress/campaign/special_interest/articles.cfm?ID=653
7

[300] The Center for Public Integrity. Drug Lobby Second to None: How the pharmaceutical industry gets its way in Washington. July 7, 2005.

www.public-i.org/rx/report.aspx?aid=723&sid=200

[301] The Center for Public Integrity. A Timeline of Political Clout: Here's what the pharmaceutical industry has gotten on its political investment.

www.public-i.org/rx/report.aspx?aid=719

[302] Testimony of Sidney M. Wolfe, MD, Director, Public Citizen's Health Research Group to Senate Commerce Committee Subcommittee on Consumer Affairs. Hearing on Direct-to-Consumer (DTC) Advertising, July 24, 2001.

[303] Dembner, "Public Handouts Enrich Drug Makers," The Boston Globe, April 5, 1998.

[304] National Institutes of Health, "NIH Contributions to Pharmaceutical Development," Administrative Document, February 2000

[305] Public Citizen. Letter to the Department of Health and Human Services urging that they implement and enforce the Code of Ethics for Government (HRG Publication #1516). March 22, 2000

[306] Center for Science in the Public Interest. Conflicts of Interest on COX-2 Panel. http://www.cspinet.org/new/200502251.html (accessed May 31, 2006)

[307] Willman D. Hidden Risks, Lethal Truths: Warner-Lambert won approval for Rezulin after masking the number of liver injuries in clinical studies. Los Angeles Times. June 30, 2002

[308] Willman D. Drugmaker Hires NIH Researcher. Los Angeles Times. December 7, 1998

[309] Mokhiber R. Top 100 Corporate Criminals of the Decade. http://www.corporatepredators.org/top100.html Accessed May 31, 2006.

[310] Willman, D. Waxman Queries NIH on Researcher's Ties. Los Angeles Times. December 9, 1998

[311] Willman, D. Rezulin's Effect on Heart Was Also Seen as Concern. Los Angeles Times. March 26, 2000

[312] Willman, D. Rezulin's Effect on Heart Was Also Seen as Concern. Los

Angeles Times. March 26, 2000

[313] Willman, D. Rezulin's Effect on Heart Was Also Seen as Concern. Los Angeles Times. March 26, 2000

[314] Willman, D. Hidden Risks, Lethal Truths Warner-Lambert won approval for Rezulin after masking the number of liver injuries in clinical studies. Los Angeles Times. June 30, 2002

[315] Wolfe SM. Statement before the Food and Drug Administration Endocrine and Metabolic Drugs Advisory Committee meeting advising them to withdraw troglitazone from the U.S. Market. March 26, 1999 (Public Citizen HRG Publication #1476)

[316] Willman D. Hidden Risks, Lethal Truths: Warner-Lambert won approval for Rezulin after masking the number of liver injuries in clinical studies. Los Angeles Times. June 30, 2002

[317] Willman D. Risk Was Known as FDA OKd Fatal Drug Study: Los Angeles Times March 11, 2001

[318] Ibid.

[319] The Lipid Research Clinics Coronary Primary Prevention Trial results. I. Reduction in incidence of coronary heart disease. JAMA. 1984 Jan 20;251(3):351-64.

[320] Troglitazone (Rezulin) Professional Product Labeling. Physicians' Desk Reference 52 ed. 1998 Montvale NJ:Medical Economics Company, Inc.

[321] Willman D. Hidden Risks, Lethal Truths: Warner-Lambert won approval for Rezulin after masking the number of liver injuries in clinical studies. Los Angeles Times. June 30, 2002

[322] Willman D. Hidden Risks, Lethal Truths: Warner-Lambert won approval for Rezulin after masking the number of liver injuries in clinical studies. Los Angeles Times. June 30, 2002

[323] Willman D. A Federal Researcher Who Defended a Client's Lethal Drug. Los Angeles Times. December 7, 2003

[324] Committee on Safety of Medicines. Troglitazone (Romozin) Current Problems in Pharmacovigilance 1997;23:13-16.)

[325] Food and Drug Administration Press Office, Patient Testing and Labeling Strengthened for Rezulin, December 1, 1997.

[326] Willman D. Death Toll Challenges Rezulin Safety Claim. Los Angeles Times. Thursday, March 18, 1999

[327] Willman D. Death Toll Challenges Rezulin Safety Claim. Los Angeles Times. Thursday, March 18, 1999

[328] Willman D. The Rise and Fall of the Killer Drug Rezulin. Los Angeles Times. June 4, 2000.

[329] Willman D. Fears Grow Over Delay in Removing Rezulin. Los Angeles Times. March 10, 2000

[330] Letter from Janet B. McGill to Sen. Edward M. Kennedy, as reported in Willman D. Fears Grow Over Delay in Removing Rezulin. Los Angeles Times. March 10, 2000

[331] Willman D. Hidden Risks, Lethal Truths: Warner-Lambert won approval for Rezulin after masking the number of liver injuries in clinical studies. Los Angeles Times. June 30, 2002

[332] Mokdad et al, Diabetes trends in the U.S.: 1990-1998. Diabetes Care. 2000 Sep;23(9):1278-83.

[333] Ibid.

[334] Centers for Disease Control and Prevention, National Center for Health Statistics, Division of Health Interview Statistics, data from the National Health Interview Survey.

[335] McCance DR, Ritchie CM, Kennedy L. Is HbA1 measurement superfluous in NIDDM? Diabetes Care. 1988 Jun;11(6):512-4.

[336] Brownlee M. The pathobiology of diabetic complications: a unifying mechanism. Diabetes. 2005 Jun;54(6):1615-25.

[337] Du X, Matsumura T, Edelstein D, Rossetti L, Zsengeller Z, Szabo C, Brownlee M. Inhibition of GAPDH activity by poly(ADP-ribose) polymerase activates three major pathways of hyperglycemic damage in endothelial cells. J Clin Invest. 2003 Oct;112(7):1049-57.

[338] Nishikawa T, Edelstein D, Du XL, Yamagishi S, Matsumura T, Kaneda Y, Yorek MA, Beebe D, Oates PJ, Hammes HP, Giardino I, Brownlee M. Normalizing mitochondrial superoxide production blocks three pathways of hyperglycaemic damage. Nature. 2000 Apr 13;404(6779):787-90.

[339] UKPDS 16 Overview of six years' therapy of type 2 diabetes - a progressive

disease. UKPDS Study Group. Diabetes (1995); 44: 1249-1258

[340] Yalow RS, Berson SA. Immunoassay of endogenous plasma insulin in man. 1960. Obes Res. 1996 Nov; 4(6): 583-600.

[341] Seltzer HS, Allen EW, Herron AL Jr, Brennan MT. Insulin secretion in response to glycemic stimulus: relation of delayed initial release to carbohydrate intolerance in mild diabetes mellitus. J Clin Invest. 1967 Mar; 46(3): 323-35.

[342] Findings and Recommendations from the American College of Endocrinology Conference on the Insulin Resistance Syndrome. Washington D.C., August 26, 2002.

[343] Temple RC, Carrington CA, Luzio SD, Owens DR, Schneider AE, Sobey WJ, Hales CN. Insulin deficiency in non-insulin-dependent diabetes. Lancet. 1989 Feb 11;1(8633):293-5.

[344] Temple RC, Clark PM, Nagi DK, Schneider AE, Yudkin JS, Hales CN. Radioimmunoassay may overestimate insulin in non-insulin-dependent diabetics. Clin Endocrinol (Oxf). 1990 Jun;32(6):689-93.

[345] Kahn SE, Halban PA. Release of incompletely processed proinsulin is the cause of the disproportionate proinsulinemia of NIDDM. Diabetes. 1997 Nov;46(11):1725-32.

[346] Temple RC, Clark PM, Nagi DK, Schneider AE, Yudkin JS, Hales CN. Radioimmunoassay may overestimate insulin in non-insulin-dependent diabetics. Clin Endocrinol (Oxf). 1990 Jun;32(6):689-93.

[347] GM Reaven, YD Chen, CB Hollenbeck, WH Sheu, D Ostrega and KS Polonsky. Plasma insulin, C-peptide, and proinsulin concentrations in obese and nonobese individuals with varying degrees of glucose tolerance. Journal of Clinical Endocrinology & Metabolism, Vol 76, 44-48, Copyright © 1993 by Endocrine Society

[348] Roder ME, Porte D Jr, Schwartz RS, Kahn SE. Disproportionately elevated proinsulin levels reflect the degree of impaired B cell secretory capacity in patients with noninsulin-dependent diabetes mellitus. J Clin Endocrinol Metab. 1998 Feb;83(2):604-8.

[349] Roder ME, Porte D Jr, Schwartz RS, Kahn SE. Disproportionately elevated proinsulin levels reflect the degree of impaired B cell secretory capacity in patients with noninsulin-dependent diabetes mellitus. J Clin Endocrinol Metab. 1998 Feb;83(2):604-8.

[350] Butler AE, Janson J, Bonner-Weir S, Ritzel R, Rizza RA, Butler PC. Beta-cell deficit and increased beta-cell apoptosis in humans with type 2 diabetes. Diabetes. 2003 Jan;52(1):102-10.

[351] Brownlee M. A radical explanation for glucose-induced beta cell dysfunction. J Clin Invest. 2003 Dec;112(12):1788-90.

[352] Krauss S, Zhang CY, Scorrano L, Dalgaard LT, St-Pierre J, Grey ST, Lowell BB. Superoxide-mediated activation of uncoupling protein 2 causes pancreatic beta cell dysfunction. J Clin Invest. 2003 Dec;112(12):1831-42.

[353] Kaiser N, Leibowitz G, Nesher R. Glucotoxicity and beta-cell failure in type 2 diabetes mellitus. J Pediatr Endocrinol Metab. 2003 Jan;16(1):5-22.

[354] Unger RH. Lipotoxicity in the pathogenesis of obesity-dependent NIDDM. Genetic and clinical implications. Diabetes 44:863-870, 1995.

[355] Kahn SE, Andrikopoulos S, Verchere CB. Islet amyloid. A long-recognized but underappreciated pathological feature of type 2 diabetes. Diabetes 48:241-253, 1999.

[356] Stern L, Iqbal N, Seshadri P, Chicano KL, Daily DA, McGrory J, Williams M, Gracely EJ, Samaha FF. The effects of low-carbohydrate versus conventional weight loss diets in severely obese adults: one-year follow-up of a randomized trial. Ann Intern Med. 2004 May 18;140(10):778-85.

[357] Gutierrez M, Akhavan M, Jovanovic L, Peterson CM. Utility of a short-term 25% carbohydrate diet on improving glycemic control in type 2 diabetes mellitus. J Am Coll Nutr. 1998 Dec;17(6):595-600.

[358] Parillo M, Giacco R, Ciardullo AV, Rivellese AA, Riccardi G. Does a high-carbohydrate diet have different effects in NIDDM patients treated with diet alone or hypoglycemic drugs? Diabetes Care. 1996 May;19(5):498-500.

[359] Sharman MJ, Gomez AL, Kraemer WJ, Volek JS. Very low-carbohydrate and low-fat diets affect fasting lipids and postprandial lipemia differently in overweight men. J Nutr. 2004 Apr;134(4):880-5.

[360] Volek JS, Sharman MJ, Gomez AL, DiPasquale C, Roti M, Pumerantz A, Kraemer WJ. Comparison of a very low-carbohydrate and low-fat diet on fasting lipids, LDL subclasses, insulin resistance, and postprandial lipemic responses in overweight women. J Am Coll Nutr. 2004 Apr;23(2):177-84.

[361] Nielsen JV, Jonsson E, Nilsson AK. Lasting improvement of hyperglycaemia and bodyweight: low-carbohydrate diet in type 2 diabetes--a brief report. Ups J

Med Sci. 2005;110(1):69-73.

[362] Boden G, Sargrad K, Homko C, Mozzoli M, Stein TP. Effect of a low-carbohydrate diet on appetite, blood glucose levels, and insulin resistance in obese patients with type 2 diabetes.Ann Intern Med. 2005 Mar 15;142(6):403-11.

[363] DeFronzo RA, Sherwin RS, Kraemer N. Effect of physical training on insulin action in obesity. Diabetes. 1987 Dec;36(12):1379-85.

[364] Schneider SH, Amorosa LF, Khachadurian AK, Ruderman NB. Studies on the mechanism of improved glucose control during regular exercise in type 2 (non-insulin-dependent) diabetes. Diabetologia. 1984 May;26(5):355-60.

[365] Holloszy JO, Schultz J, Kusnierkiewicz J, Hagberg JM, Ehsani AA. Effects of exercise on glucose tolerance and insulin resistance. Brief review and some preliminary results. Acta Med Scand Suppl. 1986;711:55-65. Review.

[366] Tight glycemic control made the liver more sensitive to insulin to produce glycogen Pratipanawatr T, Cusi K, Ngo P, Pratipanawatr W, Mandarino LJ, DeFronzo RA.Normalization of plasma glucose concentration by insulin therapy improves insulin-stimulated glycogen synthesis in type 2 diabetes. Diabetes. 2002 Feb;51(2):462-8.

[367] Vague P, Moulin JP. The defective glucose sensitivity of the B cell in non insulin dependent diabetes. Improvement after twenty hours of normoglycaemia. Metabolism. 1982 Feb;31(2):139-42.

[368] Juang JH, Wang PW, Huang MJ. Effect of dietary therapy on pancreatic beta cell function in noninsulin-dependent diabetes mellitus. J Formos Med Assoc. 1990 Aug;89(8):672-6

[369] Kosaka K, Kuzuya T, Akanuma Y, Hagura R.Increase in insulin response after treatment of overt maturity-onset diabetes is independent of the mode of treatment. Diabetologia. 1980 Jan;18(1):23-8.

[370] Clauson P, Alvarsson M, Grill V.Enhancement of B-cell secretion by blood glucose normalization in type 2 diabetes is associated with fasting C-peptide levels. J Intern Med. 1997 Jun;241(6):493-500.

[371] Maedler K, Sergeev P, Ris F, Oberholzer J, Joller-Jemelka HI, Spinas GA, Kaiser N, Halban PA, Donath MY. Glucose-induced beta cell production of IL-1beta contributes to glucotoxicity in human pancreatic islets. J Clin Invest. 2002 Sep;110(6):851-60.

[372] Farvid MS, Siassi F, Jalali M, Hosseini M, Saadat N. The impact of vitamin and/or mineral supplementation on lipid profiles in type 2 diabetes. Diabetes Res Clin Pract. 2004 Jul;65(1):21-8.

[373] Park HS, Lee YM. Effect of vitamin C supplementation on blood sugar and antioxidative status in types II diabetes mellitus patients. Taehan Kanho Hakhoe Chi. 2003 Apr;33(2):170-8.

[374] Ford ES. Vitamin supplement use and diabetes mellitus incidence among adults in the United States. Am J Epidemiol. 2001 May 1;153(9):892-7.

[375] Mangoni AA, Sherwood RA, Asonganyi B, Swift CG, Thomas S, Jackson SH. Short-term oral folic acid supplementation enhances endothelial function in patients with type 2 diabetes. Am J Hypertens. 2005 Feb;18(2 Pt 1):220-6.

[376] Lal J, Vasudev K, Kela AK, Jain SK. Effect of oral magnesium supplementation on the lipid profile and blood glucose of patients with type 2 diabetes mellitus. J Assoc Physicians India. 2003 Jan;51:37-42.

[377] Sharma A, Kharb S, Chugh SN, Kakkar R, Singh GP. Evaluation of oxidative stress before and after control of glycemia and after vitamin E supplementation in diabetic patients. Metabolism. 2000 Feb;49(2):160-2.

[378] Bursell SE, Clermont AC, Aiello LP, Aiello LM, Schlossman DK, Feener EP, Laffel L, King GL.   High-dose vitamin E supplementation normalizes retinal blood flow and creatinine clearance in patients with type 1 diabetes. Diabetes Care. 1999 Aug;22(8):1245-51.

[379] Tutuncu NB, Bayraktar M, Varli K. Reversal of defective nerve conduction with vitamin E supplementation in type 2 diabetes: a preliminary study. Diabetes Care. 1998 Nov;21(11):1915-8.

[380] Lima Mde L, Cruz T, Pousada JC, Rodrigues LE, Barbosa K, Cangucu V.   The effect of magnesium supplementation in increasing doses on the control of type 2 diabetes. Diabetes Care. 1998 May;21(5):682-6.

[381] Eriksson J, Kohvakka A. Magnesium and ascorbic acid supplementation in diabetes mellitus. Ann Nutr Metab. 1995;39(4):217-23.

[382] Robertson RP, Harmon J, Tran PO, Poitout V.   Beta-cell glucose toxicity, lipotoxicity, and chronic oxidative stress in type 2 diabetes. Diabetes. 2004 Feb;53 Suppl 1:S119-24. Review.

[383] Nishikawa T, Edelstein D, Du XL, Yamagishi S, Matsumura T, Kaneda Y, Yorek MA, Beebe D, Oates PJ, Hammes HP, Giardino I, Brownlee M.

Normalizing mitochondrial superoxide production blocks three pathways of hyperglycaemic damage. Nature. 2000 Apr 13;404(6779):787-90.

[384] Dincer Y, Akcay T, Alademir Z, Ilkova H. Effect of oxidative stress on glutathione pathway in red blood cells from patients with insulin-dependent diabetes mellitus. Metabolism. 2002 Oct;51(10):1360-2.

[385] D Giugliano, A Ceriello and G Paolisso. Oxidative stress and diabetic vascular complications. Diabetes Care, Vol 19, Issue 3 257-267, 1996.

[386] Brownlee M. Biochemistry and molecular cell biology of diabetic complications. Nature. 2001 Dec 13;414(6865):813-20.

[387] Ruhe RC, McDonald RB. Use of antioxidant nutrients in the prevention and treatment of type 2 diabetes. J Am Coll Nutr. 2001 Oct;20(5 Suppl):363S-369S;

[388] Opara EC. Role of oxidative stress in the etiology of type 2 diabetes and the effect of antioxidant supplementation on glycemic control. J Investig Med. 2004 Jan;52(1):19-23.

[389] Chowienczyk PJ, Brett SE, Gopaul NK, Meeking D, Marchetti M, Russell-Jones DL, Anggard EE, Ritter JM. Oral treatment with an antioxidant (raxofelast) reduces oxidative stress and improves endothelial function in men with type II diabetes.Diabetologia. 2000 Aug;43(8):974-7.

[390] Losonczy KG, Harris TB, Havlik RS: Vitamin E and vitamin C supplement use and risk of all cause and coronary heart disease mortality in older persons: the Established Population for Epidemiologic Studies of the Elderly. *Am J Clin Nutr* 64:190–196, 1996.

[391] Rimm EB, Stampfer MJ, Ascherio A, GioVannucci E, Colditz GA, Willett WC: Vitamin E consumption and the risk of coronary heart disease in men. N Engl J Med 328:1450–1456, 1993.

[392] Montonen J, Knekt P, Jarvinen R, Reunanen A. Dietary antioxidant intake and risk of type 2 diabetes. Diabetes Care. 2004 Feb;27(2):362-6.

[393] Sanchez-Lugo L, Mayer-Davis EJ, Howard G, Selby JV, Ayad MF, Rewers M, Haffner S: Insulin sensitivity and intake of vitamins E and C in African American, Hispanic, and non-Hispanic white men and women: the Insulin Resistance and Atherosclerosis Study (IRAS). Am J Clin Nutr 66:1224–1231, 1997.

[394] Yusuf S, Dagenais G, Pogue J, Bosch J, Sleight P: Vitamin E supplementation and cardiovascular events in high-risk patients: the Heart

Outcomes Prevention Evaluation Study Investigators. N Engl J Med 342:154–160, 2000.

[395] Mayer-Davis EJ, Bell KA, Reboussin BA, Rushing J, Marshall JA, Hamman RF: Antioxidant nutrient intake and diabetic retinopathy: the San Luis Valley Diabetes Study. Ophthalmology 105:2264–2270, 1998.

[396] Yusuf S, Dagenais G, Pogue J, Bosch J, Sleight P. Vitamin E supplementation and cardiovascular events in high-risk patients. The Heart Outcomes Prevention Evaluation Study Investigators. N Engl J Med. 2000 Jan 20;342(3):154-60.

[397] Gomez-Perez FJ, Valles-Sanchez VE, Lopez-Alvarenga JC, Choza-Romero R, Ibarra Pascuali JJ, Gonzalez Orellana R, Perez Ortiz OB, Rodriguez Padilla EG, Aguilar Salinas CA, Rull JA. Vitamin E modifies neither fructosamine nor HbA1c levels in poorly controlled diabetes. Rev Invest Clin. 1996 Nov-Dec;48(6):421-4.

[398] Chugh SN, Kakkar R, Kalra S, Sharma A. An evaluation of oxidative stress in diabetes mellitus during uncontrolled and controlled state and after vitamin E supplementation. J Assoc Physicians India. 1999 Apr;47(4):380-3.

[399] Paolisso G, D'Amore A, Galzerano D, Balbi V, Giugliano D, Varricchio M, D'Onofrio F. Daily vitamin E supplements improve metabolic control but not insulin secretion in elderly type II diabetic patients. Diabetes Care. 1993 Nov;16(11):1433-7.

[400] Paolisso G, D'Amore A, Giugliano D, Ceriello A, Varricchio M, D'Onofrio F. Pharmacologic doses of vitamin E improve insulin action in healthy subjects and non-insulin-dependent diabetic patients.Am J Clin Nutr. 1993 May;57(5):650-6.

[401] Ceriello A, Giugliano D, Quatraro A, Donzella C, Dipalo G, Lefebvre PJ. Vitamin E reduction of protein glycosylation in diabetes. New prospect for prevention of diabetic complications? Diabetes Care. 1991 Jan;14(1):68-72.

[402] Bursell SE, Clermont AC, Aiello LP, Aiello LM, Schlossman DK, Feener EP, Laffel L, King GL. High-dose vitamin E supplementation normalizes retinal blood flow and creatinine clearance in patients with type 1 diabetes. Diabetes Care. 1999 Aug;22(8):1245-51.

[403] Tutuncu NB, Bayraktar M, Varli K. Reversal of defective nerve conduction with vitamin E supplementation in type 2 diabetes: a preliminary study. Diabetes Care. 1998 Nov;21(11):1915-8.

[404] The Diabetes Control and Complications Trial Research Group. The relationship of glycemic exposure (HbA 1c) to the risk of development and progression of retinopathy in the Diabetes Control and Complications Trial. Diabetes 1995; 44: 968–83.

[405] UK Prospective Diabetes Study (UKPDS) Group. Intensive blood-glucose control with sulphonylureas or insulin compared with conventional treatment and risk of complications in patients with type 2 diabetes (UKPDS 33). Lancet 1998; 352: 837–53.

[406] Babaei-Jadidi R, Karachalias N, Ahmed N, Battah S, Thornalley PJ. Prevention of incipient diabetic nephropathy by high-dose thiamine and benfotiamine. Diabetes. 2003 Aug;52(8):2110-20.

[407] Hammes HP, Du X, Edelstein D, Taguchi T, Matsumura T, Ju Q, Lin J, Bierhaus A, Nawroth P, Hannak D, Neumaier M, Bergfeld R, Giardino I, Brownlee M. Benfotiamine blocks three major pathways of hyperglycemic damage and prevents experimental diabetic retinopathy. Nat Med. 2003 Mar;9(3):294-9.

[408] Negrisanu G, Rosu M, Bolte B, Lefter D, Dabelea D. Effects of 3-month treatment with the antioxidant alpha-lipoic acid in diabetic peripheral neuropathy. Rom J Intern Med. 1999 Jul-Sep;37(3):297-306.

[409] Tankova T, Koev D, Dakovska L. Alpha-lipoic acid in the treatment of autonomic diabetic neuropathy (controlled, randomized, open-label study). Rom J Intern Med. 2004;42(2):457-64.

[410] Ziegler D, Hanefeld M, Ruhnau KJ, Meissner HP, Lobisch M, Schutte K, Gries FA: Treatment of symptomatic diabetic peripheral neuropathy with the anti-oxidant alpha-lipoic acid. A 3-week multicentre randomized controlled trial (ALADIN Study). Diabetol 38: 1425–1433, 1995.

[411] Ziegler D, Hanefeld M, Ruhnau KJ, et al. Treatment of symptomatic diabetic polyneuropathy with the antioxidant alpha-lipoic acid: a 7-month multicenter randomized controlled trial (ALADIN III Study). ALADIN III Study Group. Alpha-Lipoic Acid in Diabetic Neuropathy. Diabetes Care. 1999;22(8):1296-1301.

[412] Jacob S, Ruus P, Hermann R, Tritschler HJ, Maerker E, Renn W, Augustin HJ, Dietze GJ, Rett K. Oral administration of RAC-alpha-lipoic acid modulates insulin sensitivity in patients with type-2 diabetes mellitus: a placebo-controlled

pilot trial. Free Radic Biol Med. 1999 Aug;27(3-4):309-14.

[413] Rett K, Wicklmayr E, Maerker P, Russ D, Nehrdich D, Hermann R. Effect of acute infusion of thioctic acid on oxidative and non-oxidative metabolism in obese subjects with NIDDM. Diabetologia. 1995;38:A41.

[414] Jacob S, Henriksen EJ, Schiemann AL, et al. Enhancement of glucose disposal in patients with type 2 diabetes by alpha-lipoic acid. Arzneimittelforschung. 1995;45(8):872-874.

[415] Eibl NL, Kopp HP, Nowak HR, Schnack CJ, Hopmeier PG, Schernthaner G. Hypomagnesemia in type II diabetes: effect of a 3-month replacement therapy. Diabetes Care. 1995 Feb;18(2):188-92.

[416] Lima Mde L, Cruz T, Pousada JC, Rodrigues LE, Barbosa K, Cangucu V. The effect of magnesium supplementation in increasing doses on the control of type 2 diabetes. Diabetes Care. 1998 May;21(5):682-6.

[417] Anderson RA, Cheng N, Bryden NA, Polansky MM, Cheng N, Chi J, Feng J. Elevated intakes of supplemental chromium improve glucose and insulin variables in individuals with type 2 diabetes. Diabetes. 1997 Nov;46(11):1786-91.

[418] Bahijiri SM, Mira SA, Mufti AM, Ajabnoor MA. The effects of inorganic chromium and brewer's yeast supplementation on glucose tolerance, serum lipids and drug dosage in individuals with type 2 diabetes. Saudi Med J. 2000 Sep;21(9):831-7.

[419] Anderson RA, Roussel AM, Zouari N, Mahjoub S, Matheau JM, Kerkeni A. Potential antioxidant effects of zinc and chromium supplementation in people with type 2 diabetes mellitus. J Am Coll Nutr. 2001 Jun;20(3):212-8.

[420] Thomas VL, Gropper SS. Effect of chromium nicotinic acid supplementation on selected cardiovascular disease risk factors. Biol Trace Elem Res. 1996 Dec;55(3):297-305.

[421] Lee NA, Reasner CA. Beneficial effect of chromium supplementation on serum triglyceride levels in NIDDM. Diabetes Care. 1994 Dec;17(12):1449-52.

[422] Abraham AS, Brooks BA, Eylath U. The effects of chromium supplementation on serum glucose and lipids in patients with and without non-insulin-dependent diabetes. Metabolism. 1992 Jul;41(7):768-71.

[423] Anderson RA, Kozlovsky AS: Chromium intake, absorption and excretion of subjects consuming self-selected diets. Am J Clin Nutr 41: 1177–1183, 1985.

[424] Rajpathak S, Rimm EB, Li T, Morris JS, Stampfer MJ, Willett WC, Hu FB. Lower toenail chromium in men with diabetes and cardiovascular disease compared with healthy men. Diabetes Care. 2004 Sep;27(9):2211-6.

[425] Boden G, Chen X, Ruiz J, van Rossum GD, Turco S. Effects of vanadyl sulfate on carbohydrate and lipid metabolism in patients with non-insulin-dependent diabetes mellitus. Metabolism. 1996 Sep;45(9):1130-5.

[426] Halberstam M, Cohen N, Shlimovich P, Rossetti L, Shamoon H. Oral vanadyl sulfate improves insulin sensitivity in NIDDM but not in obese nondiabetic subjects. Diabetes. 1996 May;45(5):659-66. Erratum in: Diabetes 1996 Sep;45(9):1285.

[427] Cohen N, Halberstam M, Shlimovich P, Chang CJ, Shamoon H, Rossetti L. Oral vanadyl sulfate improves hepatic and peripheral insulin sensitivity in patients with non-insulin-dependent diabetes mellitus. J Clin Invest. 1995 Jun;95(6):2501-9.

[428] Goldfine AB, Simonson DC, Folli F, Patti ME, Kahn CR. Metabolic effects of sodium metavanadate in humans with insulin-dependent and noninsulin-dependent diabetes mellitus in vivo and in vitro studies. J Clin Endocrinol Metab. 1995 Nov;80(11):3311-20.

[429] Goldfine AB, Patti ME, Zuberi L, Goldstein BJ, LeBlanc R, Landaker EJ, Jiang ZY, Willsky GR, Kahn CR. Metabolic effects of vanadyl sulfate in humans with non-insulin-dependent diabetes mellitus: in vivo and in vitro studies. Metabolism. 2000 Mar;49(3):400-10.

[430] Cusi K, Cukier S, DeFronzo RA, Torres M, Puchulu FM, Redondo JC. Vanadyl sulfate improves hepatic and muscle insulin sensitivity in type 2 diabetes. J Clin Endocrinol Metab. 2001 Mar;86(3):1410-7.

[431] Giancaterini A, De Gaetano A, Mingrone G, Gniuli D, Liverani E, Capristo E, Greco AV: Acetyl-L-carnitine infusion increases glucose disposal in type 2 diabetic patients. Metabolism 49:704–708, 2000

[432] Mingrone G, Greco AV, Capristo E, Benedetti G, Giancaterini A, De Gaetano A, Gasbarrini G: L-carnitine improves glucose disposal in type 2 diabetic patients. J Am Coll Nutr 18:77–82, 1999

[433] Capaldo B, Napoli R, Di Bonito P, Albano G, Sacca: L Carnitine improves peripheral glucose disposal in non-insulin-dependent diabetic patients. Diabetes Res Clin Pract 14:191–195, 1991

[434] Harper P, Elwin C-E, Cederblad G: Pharmacokinetics of bolus intravenous and oral doses of L-carnitine in healthy subjects. Eur J Clin Pharmacol 35: 69–75, 1988.

[435] Brass EP, Hiatt WR. The role of carnitine and carnitine supplementation during exercise in man and in individuals with special needs. J Am Coll Nutr. 1998;17(3):207-215.

[436] Azad Khan AK, Akhtar S, Mahtab H. Coccinia indica in the treatment of patients with diabetes mellitus. Bangladesh Med Res Counc Bull. 1979 Dec;5(2):60-6.

[437] Kamble SM, Jyotishi GS, Kamlakar PL, Vaidya SM. Efficacy of *Coccinia indica* W.& A in diabetes mellitus. J Res Ayurveda Siddha. XVII:77-84, 1996.

[438] Kamble SM, Kamlakar PL, Vaidya S, Bambole VD. Influence of Coccinia indica on certain enzymes in glycolytic and lipolytic pathway in human diabetes. Indian J Med Sci. 1998 Apr;52(4):143-6.

[439] Sitprija S, Plengvidhya C, Kangkaya V, Bhuvapanich S, Tunkayoon M. Garlic and diabetes mellitus phase II clinical trial. J Med Assoc Thai. 1987 Mar;70 Suppl 2:223-7.

[440] Sharma RD, Raghuram TC. Hypoglycemic effect of fenugreek seeds in non-insulin dependent diabetic subjects. Nutr Res 10:731-739, 1990.

[441] Madar Z, Abel R, Samish S, Arad J. Glucose-lowering effect of fenugreek in non-insulin dependent diabetics. Eur J Clin Nutr. 1988 Jan;42(1):51-4.

[442] Gupta A, Gupta R, Lal B. Effect of Trigonella foenum-graecum (fenugreek) seeds on glycaemic control and insulin resistance in type 2 diabetes mellitus: a double blind placebo controlled study. J Assoc Physicians India. 2001 Nov;49:1057-61.

[443] Agrawal P, Rai V, Singh RB. Randomized placebo-controlled, single blind trial of holy basil leaves in patients with noninsulin-dependent diabetes mellitus. Int J Clin Pharmacol Ther. 1996 Sep;34(9):406-9.

[444] Baskaran K, Kizar Ahamath B, Radha Shanmugasundaram K, Shanmugasundaram ER. Antidiabetic effect of a leaf extract from Gymnema sylvestre in non-insulin-dependent diabetes mellitus patients. J Ethnopharmacol. 1990 Oct;30(3):295-300.

[445] Welihinda J, Karunanayake EH, Sheriff MH, Jayasinghe KS. Effect of Momordica charantia on the glucose tolerance in maturity onset diabetes. J

Ethnopharmacol. 1986 Sep;17(3):277-82.

[446] Frati-Munari AC, Gordillo BE, Altamirano P, Ariza CR. Hypoglycemic effect of Opuntia streptacantha Lemaire in NIDDM. Diabetes Care. 1988 Jan;11(1):63-6.

[447] Sotaniemi EA, Haapakoski E, Rautio A. Ginseng therapy in non-insulin-dependent diabetic patients. Diabetes Care. 1995 Oct;18(10):1373-5.

[448] Vuksan V, Stavro MP, Sievenpiper JL, Koo VY, Wong E, Beljan-Zdravkovic U, Francis T, Jenkins AL, Leiter LA, Josse RG, Xu Z.   American ginseng improves glycemia in individuals with normal glucose tolerance: effect of dose and time escalation. J Am Coll Nutr. 2000 Nov-Dec;19(6):738-44.

[449] Cui J, Garle M, Eneroth P, Bjorkhem I. What do commercial ginseng preparations contain? Lancet. 1994 Jul 9;344(8915):134.

[450] Heinemann L. Variability of insulin absorption and insulin action. Diabetes Technol Ther. 2002;4(5):673-82. Review.

[451] Pickup J, Mattock M, Kerry S. Glycaemic control with continuous subcutaneous insulin infusion compared with intensive insulin injections in patients with type 1 diabetes: meta-analysis of randomised controlled trials. BMJ. 2002 Mar 23;324(7339):705.

[452] Dunn FL, Nathan DM, Scavini M, Selam JL, Wingrove TG. Long-term therapy of IDDM with an implantable insulin pump. The Implantable Insulin Pump Trial Study Group. Diabetes Care. 1997 Jan;20(1):59-63.

[453] Renard E.   Implantable closed-loop glucose-sensing and insulin delivery: the future for insulin pump therapy. Curr Opin Pharmacol. 2002 Dec;2(6):708-16.

[454] Simonson DC, Kourides IA, Feinglos M, Shamoon H, Fischette CT. Efficacy, safety, and dose-response characteristics of glipizide gastrointestinal therapeutic system on glycemic control and insulin secretion in NIDDM. Results of two multicenter, randomized, placebo-controlled clinical trials. The Glipizide Gastrointestinal Therapeutic System Study Group.Diabetes Care. 1997 Apr;20(4):597-606.

[455] Rosenstock J, Samols E, Muchmore DB, Schneider J. Glimepiride, a new once-daily sulfonylurea. A double-blind placebo-controlled study of NIDDM patients. Glimepiride Study Group. Diabetes Care. 1996 Nov;19(11):1194-9.

[456] UK Prospective Diabetes Study (UKPDS) Group. Intensive blood-glucose

control with sulphonylureas or insulin compared with conventional treatment and risk of complications in patients with type 2 diabetes (UKPDS 33). Lancet. 1998 Sep 12;352(9131):837-53.

[457] Rustenbeck I. Desensitization of insulin secretion. Biochem Pharmacol. 2002 Jun 1;63(11):1921-35. Review.

[458] Intensive blood-glucose control with sulphonylureas or insulin compared with conventional treatment and risk of complications in patients with type 2 diabetes (UKPDS 33). UK Prospective Diabetes Study (UKPDS) Group. Lancet. 1998 Sep 12;352(9131):837-53.

[459] Intensive blood-glucose control with sulphonylureas or insulin compared with conventional treatment and risk of complications in patients with type 2 diabetes (UKPDS 33). UK Prospective Diabetes Study (UKPDS) Group. Lancet. 1998 Sep 12;352(9131):837-53.

[460] Intensive blood-glucose control with sulphonylureas or insulin compared with conventional treatment and risk of complications in patients with type 2 diabetes (UKPDS 33). UK Prospective Diabetes Study (UKPDS) Group. Lancet. 1998 Sep 12;352(9131):837-53.

[461] University Group Diabetes Program. A study of the effects of hypoglycemic agents on vascular complications in patients with adult-onset diabetes. *Diabetes* 1970; 19(suppl 2): 747-830.

[462] Rizzo MR, Barbieri M, Grella R, Passariello N, Barone M, Paolisso G. Repaglinide is more efficient than glimepiride on insulin secretion and post-prandial glucose excursions in patients with type 2 diabetes. A short term study.

[463] Cozma LS, Luzio SD, Dunseath GJ, Langendorg KW, Pieber T, Owens DR. Comparison of the effects of three insulinotropic drugs on plasma insulin levels after a standard meal. Diabetes Care. 2002 Aug;25(8):1271-6.

[464] Madsbad S, Kilhovd B, Lager I, Mustajoki P, Dejgaard A; Scandinavian Repaglinide Group. Comparison between repaglinide and glipizide in Type 2 diabetes mellitus: a 1-year multicentre study. Diabet Med. 2001 May;18(5):395-401.

[465] University Group Diabetes Program. A study of the effects of hypoglycemic agents on vascular complications in patients with adult-onset diabetes. Diabetes 1970; 19 (suppl 2): 747–830.

[466] Dr Marios Kyriazis, M.D., Bios, Cross-link Breakers and Inhibitors,

http://www.antiaging-systems.com/extract/crosslinking.htm

[467] Diabetes Prevention Research Group: Reduction in the evidence of type 2 diabetes with life-style intervention or metformin. New England Journal of Medicine 346:393-403, 2002.

[468] DeFronzo RA, Goodman AM. Efficacy of metformin in patients with non-insulin-dependent diabetes mellitus. The Multicenter Metformin Study Group. N Engl J Med. 1995 Aug 31;333(9):541-9.

[469] UK Prospective Diabetes Study (UKPDS) Group. Effect of intensive blood-glucose control with metformin on complications in overweight patients with type 2 diabetes (UKPDS 34). Lancet. 1998 Sep 12;352(9131):854-65.

[470] UK Prospective Diabetes Study (UKPDS) Group. Effect of intensive blood-glucose control with metformin on complications in overweight patients with type 2 diabetes (UKPDS 34). Lancet. 1998 Sep 12;352(9131):854-65.

[471] Sum CF, Webster JM, Johnson AB, Catalano C, Cooper BG, Taylor R. The effect of intravenous metformin on glucose metabolism during hyperglycaemia in type 2 diabetes. Diabet Med. 1992 Jan-Feb;9(1):61-5.

[472] Bailey CJ. Metformin: a useful adjunct to insulin therapy? Diabet Med. 2000 Jan;17(1):83-4.

[473] Bailey CJ, Turner RC. Metformin. N Engl J Med 1996;334:574-9.

[474] Reduction of glycosylated hemoglobin and postprandial hyperglycemia by acarbose in patients with NIDDM. A placebo-controlled dose-comparison study. Diabetes Care. 1995 Jun;18(6):817-24.

[475] Chiasson JL, Josse RG, Hunt JA, Palmason C, Rodger NW, Ross SA, Ryan EA, Tan MH, Wolever TM. The efficacy of acarbose in the treatment of patients with non-insulin-dependent diabetes mellitus. A multicenter controlled clinical trial. Ann Intern Med. 1994 Dec 15;121(12):928-35.

[476] Scott LJ, Spencer CM. Miglitol: a review of its therapeutic potential in type 2 diabetes mellitus. Drugs 2000;59:512-49.

[477] Haluzik M, Parizkova J, Haluzik MM. Adiponectin and its role in the obesity-induced insulin resistance and related complications. Physiol Res. 2004;53(2):123-9.

[478] Yang X, Jansson PA, Nagaev I, Jack MM, Carvalho E, Sunnerhagen KS, Cam MC, Cushman SW, Smith U. Evidence of impaired adipogenesis in insulin

resistance. Biochem Biophys Res Commun. 2004 May 14;317(4):1045-51.

[479] Chen XP, Yang WY, Bu S, Xiao JZ, Liu XL, Wang N, Zhao WH. [Effects of rosiglitazone and metformin on insulin resistance in high-fat diet rats] Zhonghua Nei Ke Za Zhi. 2004 Apr;43(4):280-3. Chinese.

[480] Maggs DG, Buchanan TA, Burant CF, Cline G, Gumbiner B, Hsueh WA, Inzucchi S, Kelley D, Nolan J, Olefsky JM, Polonsky KS, Silver D, Valiquett TR, Shulman GI. Metabolic effects of troglitazone monotherapy in type 2 diabetes mellitus. A randomized, double-blind, placebo-controlled trial. Ann Intern Med. 1998 Feb 1;128(3):176-85.

[481] Mudaliar S, Chang AR, Henry RR. Thiazolidinediones, peripheral edema, and type 2 diabetes: incidence, pathophysiology, and clinical implications. ndocr Pract. 2003 Sep-Oct;9(5):406-16. Review.

[482] Wooltorton E. Rosiglitazone (Avandia) and pioglitazone (Actos) and heart failure. CMAJ. 2002 Jan 22;166(2):219.

[483] Kermani A, Garg A.   Thiazolidinedione-associated congestive heart failure and pulmonary edema. Mayo Clin Proc. 2003 Sep;78(9):1088-91

[484] Delea TE, Edelsberg JS, Hagiwara M, et al. Use of thiazolidinediones and risk of heart failure in people with type 2 diabetes. Diabetes Care 2003; 26:2983-2989.

[485] Marcy TR, Britton ML, Blevins SM. Second-generation thiazolidinediones and hepatotoxicity. Ann Pharmacother. 2004 Sep;38(9):1419-23. Epub 2004 Jul 20.

[486] Farilla L, Bulotta A, Hirshberg B, Li Calzi S, Khoury N, Noushmehr H, Bertolotto C, Di Mario U, Harlan DM, Perfetti R. GLP-1 inhibits cell apoptosis and improves glucose responsiveness of freshly isolated human islets. Endocrinology. 2003 Aug 28.

[487] Farilla L, Bulotta A, Hirshberg B, Li Calzi S, Khoury N, Noushmehr H, Bertolotto C, Di Mario U, Harlan DM, Perfetti R.GLP-1 inhibits cell apoptosis and improves glucose responsiveness of freshly isolated human islets. Endocrinology. 2003 Aug 28

[488] Buteau J, Foisy S, Joly E, Prentki M Glucagon-like peptide 1 induces pancreatic beta-cell proliferation via transactivation of the epidermal growth factor receptor. Diabetes. 2003 Jan;52(1):124-32

[489] Ahren B, Holst JJ, Mari A. Characterization of GLP-1 effects on beta-cell

function after meal ingestion in humans. Diabetes Care. 2003 Oct;26(10):2860-4.

[490] Rosenberg L, Duguid WP, Brown RA, Vinik AI. Induction of nesidioblastosis will reverse diabetes in Syrian golden hamster. Diabetes. 1988 Mar;37(3):334-41.

[491] Mayers D. Would You Cure A Profitable Disease? Diabetes Health, October 2003

[492] Update on Islet Regeneration Research – SPIRIT Team Pushing Forward With Positive Results From Phase 2 Trials http://www.dif.org/n_articles/ingapupdate.html Accessed July 20, 2006

[493] Update on Islet Regeneration Research – SPIRIT Team Pushing Forward With Positive Results From Phase 2 Trials http://www.dif.org/n_articles/ingapupdate.html Accessed July 20, 2006

[494] Mendosa, David. The INGAP Revival. Tuesday, May 30th, 2006. http://blogs.healthcentral.com/diabetes/david-mendosa/the-ingap-revival-2006-05-30 accessed July 20, 2006.

[495] Jiang R, Manson JE, Stampfer MJ, Liu S, Willett WC, Hu FB. Nut and peanut butter consumption and risk of type 2 diabetes in women. JAMA. 2002 Nov 27;288(20):2554-60.

[496] Hites RA, Foran JA, Carpenter DO, Hamilton MC, Knuth BA, Schwager SJ. Global assessment of organic contaminants in farmed salmon. Science. 2004 Jan 9;303(5655):226-9.

[497] Wal JM. Bovine milk allergenicity.Ann Allergy Asthma Immunol. 2004 Nov;93(5 Suppl 3):S2-11.

[498] Host A. Frequency of cow's milk allergy in childhood. Ann Allergy Asthma Immunol. 2002 Dec;89(6 Suppl 1):33-7.

[499] Douglass William Campbell, MD: The Milk Book, The Milk of Human Kindness is not Pasteurized. Rhino Publishing. ISBN 9962-636-54-X

[500] The Campaign for Real Milk. http://www.realmilk.com/

[501] Schmid Ron, ND, The Untold Story of Milk : Green Pastures, Contented Cows and Raw Dairy Products. NewTrends Publishing, Inc. 2005. ISBN: 0967089743

[502] Hu FB, Stampfer MJ, Rimm EB, Manson JE, Ascherio A, Colditz GA,

Rosner BA, Spiegelman D, Speizer FE, Sacks FM, Hennekens CH, Willett WC. A prospective study of egg consumption and risk of cardiovascular disease in men and women. JAMA. 1999 Apr 21;281(15):1387-94.

[503] Keijzers GB, De Galan BE, Tack CJ, Smits P. Caffeine can decrease insulin sensitivity in humans. Diabetes Care. 2002;25:364-9.

[504] Feinberg LJ, Sandberg H, De Castro O, Bellet S. Effects of coffee ingestion on oral glucose tolerance curves in normal human subjects. Metabolism. 1968; 17:916-22.

[505] Agardh EE, Carlsson S, Ahlbom A, Efendic S, Grill V, Hammar N, Hilding A, Ostenson CG. Coffee consumption, type 2 diabetes and impaired glucose tolerance in Swedish men and women. J Intern Med. 2004 Jun;255(6):645-52.

[506] van Dam RM, Dekker JM, Nijpels G, Stehouwer CD, Bouter LM, Heine RJ. Coffee consumption and incidence of impaired fasting glucose, impaired glucose tolerance, and type 2 diabetes: the Hoorn Study. Diabetologia. 2004 Dec;47(12):2152-9. Epub 2004 Dec 11.

[507] Tuomilehto J, Hu G, Bidel S, Lindstrom J, Jousilahti P. Coffee consumption and risk of type 2 diabetes mellitus among middle-aged Finnish men and women. JAMA. 2004 Mar 10;291(10):1213-9

[508] Salazar-Martinez E, Willett WC, Ascherio A, Manson JE, Leitzmann MF, Stampfer MJ, Hu FB. Coffee consumption and risk for type 2 diabetes mellitus. Ann Intern Med. 2004 Jan 6;140(1):1-8.

[509] Yamaji T, Mizoue T, Tabata S, Ogawa S, Yamaguchi K, Shimizu E, Mineshita M, Kono S. Coffee consumption and glucose tolerance status in middle-aged Japanese men. Diabetologia. 2004 Dec;47(12):2145-51. Epub 2004 Dec 15.

[510] Howard AA, Arnsten JH, Gourevitch MN. Effect of alcohol consumption on diabetes mellitus: a systematic review. Ann Intern Med. 2004 Feb 3;140(3):211-9.

[511] Sierksma A, Patel H, Ouchi N, Kihara S, Funahashi T, Heine RJ, Grobbee DE, Kluft C, Hendriks HF. Effect of moderate alcohol consumption on adiponectin, tumor necrosis factor-alpha, and insulin sensitivity. Diabetes Care. 2004 Jan;27(1):184-9.

[512] Avogaro A, Watanabe RM, Dall'Arche A, De Kreutzenberg SV, Tiengo A, Pacini G. Acute alcohol consumption improves insulin action without affecting

insulin secretion in type 2 diabetic subjects. Diabetes Care. 2004
Jun;27(6):1369-74.

[513] Scragg R, Metcalf P. Do triglycerides explain the U-shaped relation between
alcohol and diabetes risk? Results from a cross-sectional survey of alcohol and
plasma glucose. Diabetes Res Clin Pract. 2004 Nov;66(2):147-56.

[514] Howard AA, Arnsten JH, Gourevitch MN. Effect of alcohol consumption on
diabetes mellitus: a systematic review. Ann Intern Med. 2004 Feb 3;140(3):211-
9.

www.ingramcontent.com/pod-product-compliance
Lightning Source LLC
Chambersburg PA
CBHW030256290526
45785CB00001B/103